TO THE RESCUE

Stories from Healthcare Workers at the Scenes of Disasters

TO THE RESCUE

Stories from Healthcare Workers at the Scenes of Disasters

Nancy Leigh Harless, ARNP
Kerry-Ann Morris
Editors

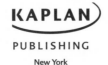

PUBLISHING

New York

© 2009 Nancy Leigh Harless and Kerry-Ann Morris

Published by Kaplan Publishing, a division of Kaplan, Inc.
1 Liberty Plaza, 24th Floor
New York, NY 10006

Library of Congress Cataloging-in-Publication Data

To the rescue : stories from healthcare workers at the scene of disaster / [edited by] Nancy Leigh Harless, Kerry-Ann Morris.

p. ; cm.

ISBN 978-1-4277-9972-2

1. Disaster medicine. 2. Medical emergencies. 3. Rescue work. I. Harless, Nancy Leigh. II. Morris, Kerry-Ann.

[DNLM: 1. Health Personnel--psychology--Personal Narratives. 2. Disasters--Personal Narratives. WZ 112 T627 2009]

RC86.7.T6 2009

363.34'8--dc22

2009014045

Printed in the United States of America

10 9 8 7 6 5 4 3 2 1

ISBN: 978-1-4277-9972-2

Kaplan Publishing books are available at special quantity discounts to use for sales promotions, employee premiums, or educational purposes. Please email our Special Sales Department to order or for more information at *kaplanpublishing@kaplan.com*, or write to Kaplan Publishing, 1 Liberty Plaza, 24th Floor, New York, NY 10006.

Contents

Introduction: Out of Tragedy Comes Resilience

ON SEPTEMBER 11, 2001, the world bore witness to the worst terrorist attack ever to occur on U.S. soil. Today "9/11" is synonymous with that World Trade Center tragedy. For those who worked at the forefront of the emergency response at Ground Zero, memories of dust, destroyed lives, and tired yet resolute firefighters rescuing and interacting with survivors will forever come to mind.

Healthcare professionals are on the front lines of all types of disasters and are expected to respond quickly and effectively to many kinds of emergencies—more so now than at any time in our immediate history. Every year, more than 200 million people are affected by droughts, floods, cyclones, earthquakes, and other natural hazards. Increased population densities, environmental degradation, and global warming, in addition to poverty, make the impacts of natural hazards worse. In the past few years, we have been reminded of the magnitude of the effects of natural hazards. From the Indian Ocean tsunami to the devastation caused by hurricanes and cyclones in the United States and the Caribbean, hundreds of thousands of people have lost their lives, and millions their livelihoods, to disasters caused by natural hazards.

With this increase in worldwide disasters, both natural and man-made, the role of the emergency healthcare professional has become even more important. Recognizing this importance will make a difference in how helpful one can be to the victims of such disasters. Emergency healthcare workers will be more effective at their jobs during a disaster if they believe it is important for them to work under crisis conditions—not only for the victims, but for themselves as human beings. In one of the essays in this volume, "There Is a Way from Heart to Heart," the passion Jeffery Goodman brings to bear on the lives of those affected by crises made a difference not only in the lives he touched but in his own life as well. He was able to find his "own inner strength and resilience and the inspiration to move forward and discover deep fulfillment in loss."

To the Rescue presents a plethora of stories by healthcare workers from a variety of specialties, including EMTs, doctors, mental health specialists and nurses, who have gone to the scenes of disasters in their hometowns and across the world. These stories illustrate the resilience of the human spirit in the face of so much tragedy and the ways one can learn from loss. People have the positive capacity to cope with stress and catastrophe. They not only recover, but can even grow through adversity. In

"Beauty and Grace," Grace Muthumbi touches on personal disasters as positive and transformative experiences that help to heal others who face their own personal disasters. This is further explored in Mark Montijo's "Hunting the Lion That Swallowed You," in which we are urged to embrace trauma as our teacher and discern meaning from the experience in order to make sense of our realities and become stronger and more resilient.

The lesson of resilience applies to everyone: victims and disaster workers alike. Linda Garrett learns this truth while working in the post–hurricane Katrina recovery effort. In Louisiana she meets one optimistic man, determined not to move from his storm-wrecked home, who serves her coffee—with true Southern hospitality—in mismatched cups and saucers, "the good china," scrounged from the debris of his home.

Marko Cunningham's "Tsunami!" forces one to question the sanity of choosing this career. His story is probably the most profound example of tenacity, determination, and resilience, as he recounts the physically and emotionally demanding work of recovering bodies after the tsunami in Thailand. Marko thought of many excuses he could have used to remove himself from this difficult task; but rather than quit, he reached deep inside himself for the strength to continue, a task he continues to do after the end of his story.

In each story in *To the Rescue*, we are invited to take a drive down memory lane with a disaster healthcare worker who not only recounts a disaster's impact, but also gives us a glimpse into the real-time application of the time-honored philosophy of being our brother's keeper. Even in times of war, we can help others and bring new life in the seeming darkness. This is most evident in LeAnn Thieman's "How Did I Get Myself into This?" Since childhood, she was compelled to give to others less fortunate than herself, as well as to adopt a child. Her reward for her small part in rescuing 100 babies during the Vietnam War was a son of her own.

And, of course, all these stories of disaster and tragedy bring home the theme of service. In times of disaster, many come together in a joint effort to overcome adversity and to bring back a sense of normality to those directly and indirectly affected by the tragedies. Sam Bradley's recounting of the rescue operations at Ground Zero clearly illustrates this point. As a member of the Federal Disaster Medical Assistance Team from California, Sam saw firsthand the human carnage caused by this tragedy, but was grateful for the role she played in the recovery efforts. As she states at the end of her recollection: "Some of us have lingering psychological trauma. Despite that, we were grateful and honored to have served our country and the people of New York City."

As the famous football coach Vince Lombardi once said: "People who work together will win, whether it be against complex football defenses, or the problems of modern society." Vince could have been speaking about disaster workers and the teamwork involved in emergency work. In two separate stories of flood disasters from opposite sides of the world, contributors Chad Ware of Iowa and Julie Vickery of New Zealand credit their staff with the success in maintaining healthcare to patients during severe floods. In both stories, members of their staffs pulled together and used extraordinary means to provide for their patients. Ware and Vickery sing the praises of their workers' dedication and sense of camaraderie.

How can one try to prevent a disaster from becoming a personal tragedy? Try laughing. This is explored in "Clowns to the Rescue" by Dionetta Hudzinski, a nurse who works primarily with people who are in pain and dying. Hudzinski, along with her clown contingent from all over the United States, "gathered in New York City to bring hope and laughter as New Yorkers faced the anniversary of the 9/11 tragedy." Instead of being shunned by the New Yorkers they met on their tour, they were welcomed and encouraged to "clown around." They brought laughter to New York on the somber occasion of the first anniversary of the World Trade Center attack.

Other methods include talking and writing. Disasters, natural or man-made, are jarring to our sense of safety. Survivors have the fundamental need to tell their personal, unique story. It is just as important that their story be heard, truly heard, and that their experiences be thereby validated. Perry Prince was all too aware of the need for telling one's story. In "The Day of the Great Wave," Prince encourages a group of tsunami survivors to use a tube of sunscreen as a "talking stick" so that each has time to speak and to listen to each other's stories.

So welcome to the memories of emergency healthcare workers in *To the Rescue*. Each recollection has a special meaning for the writer, and each has a fundamental lesson to teach us. These are just a few stories of those who willingly go to the scene of disasters to help and interact with survivors. In these recollections we witness the worst that human beings bring to each other in times of war and the impact of nature on human life; but we also witness the resilience of the human spirit and the call to serve that these individuals answer.

There Is a Way from
Heart to Heart

≈

Jeffrey C. Goodman, MD

I WAS LIVING THE good life. I had a beautiful wife and two great kids, and I lived in a place where people spend their dream vacations. Then in 1986 something happened that would change my life dramatically.

Growing up in Los Angeles, I saw how much my parents always wanted to take a vacation but never did, so I decided that I would live in a place where I would want to spend my holiday. For about 15 years, I was a small-town physician in Kilauea, Hawaii. I had a nice practice and spent my days delivering babies, performing minor surgeries, working in the emergency room, and doing all the things that doctors do.

Even in this idyllic setting I started to itch, not for another island paradise, but for the mountainous, turbulent border dividing Afghanistan and Pakistan.

My calling to the Middle East began in 1986 when Dan Rather produced a television special on the plight of the Afghan people during the Soviet invasion, in which he actually entered Afghanistan with the Mujahideen. Like everyone, I had followed the Soviet invasion of Afghanistan and the cancellation of the Olympics, but none of it affected me as much as this presentation.

At that time, the war had been going on for seven years. When it ended three years later, 1.3 million Afghans had lost their lives and 7.5 million had fled their homes to live in crowded refugee camps or shantytowns with little or no food, water, or shelter. Three million fled to Pakistan, where I would soon begin my long relationship with the Afghan people.

I went to bed that night, just like any other night, but I woke up at about 3:00 A.M., unusual because I'm one who sleeps well. Unable to fall back asleep, I went out on the patio and decided, right then and there, that I was going to do something for the Afghan people. I had a near-perfect life with my family in Hawaii, but I knew that it was time to give back. I went back to sleep.

The next morning I started thinking, *Now how in the heck am I going to find someone to be a vehicle for me to work with the Afghan people?*

I found that opportunity with the International Medical Corps (IMC), a small organization based in

Santa Monica, California. Over the years, IMC went on to work in more than 50 countries and to respond to some of the most devastating emergencies of our time, including the Rwandan genocide, the conflict in Darfur, the Southeast Asian tsunami, and the cyclone that hit Myanmar. Back then, it was just getting its start and had a single mission: to train Afghan medics to practice healthcare so that they could take care of their people.

At that time, 90 percent of the medical care in Afghanistan was centered in Kabul, while only 10 percent was out in the field. The Soviet invasion destroyed what little healthcare system existed, and most Afghan physicians fled the country. People were left without any access to medical care, particularly in the rural areas, where it was virtually nonexistent. IMC created a nine-month medical training program in Nasir Bagh, a refugee camp near Peshawar, along the Afghan border. The program was designed to get qualified health professionals back into the country by training Afghan refugees to practice basic healthcare. The graduating medics were then given supplies and medications to set up health clinics in their home villages and begin caring for their people.

When I decided to go to Pakistan, my children were 12 and 14 years old—too young to understand what was involved. My wife seemed proud of me: nobody we knew did this kind of work overseas. She looked at me and said, "I knew you had this in you and sometime you were going to have to go, so go do it and get it over with."

Peshawar was, and still is, a dangerous place. I was naïve about what I was getting myself into. I had never visited a developing country or put myself in the path of danger. I had my wake-up call just a few days after I got there.

I arrived in Nasir Bagh in time for the second training class, joining a group of eight or ten volunteer doctors and nurses and 24 students. Our time was divided between the classroom and the clinic, which provided on-the-job training for the students. The clinic, classrooms, and living accommodations were all inside the compound. Encircled by walls punctuated by guards at each corner, the compound was an unconcealed reminder that our work was set against a treacherous backdrop, one that could threaten our lives and the mission at any time.

The first threat happened within days of my arrival. We awoke to a huge explosion, the impact sending tremors throughout the compound. Someone had thrown a grenade over the wall, sending debris like confetti into the air. The classroom windows shattered. Shrapnel hit one of our guards in the neck. Our surgeon repaired the guard's injuries and there were no casualties, but the experience had been unsettling. We knew it was a direct attack on us. Suddenly, the danger of what we were doing became very real.

Two days later, I was giving a lecture in the class with the broken windows when another blast rocked the compound. I paused, my hand still holding a piece of chalk to the blackboard, and turned around to look at my students. They looked at one another with wide, concerned eyes. We all knew what had happened. We recognized the sound of bombs, the deafening thump they make when they go off, like a book falling onto an oak table.

I did not stop the lecture. I just kept right on going as if nothing had happened. None of the students interrupted or left the classroom to see what was going on. We finished the lesson together, determined not to let anything get in the way. It was as if my subconscious said to me: *They are not going to stop us. We are going to continue to train these people. We have a job to do, and we're damn well going to do it.*

When the class was over, we discovered that someone had blown up a bus right in front of the compound. The bus looked like a tin can that had a cherry bomb go off inside it. The sides and roof were pushed out; all the windows broken. Three people were killed and about 20 others were injured. All the injured people were hustled into our clinic and treated, something that may never have happened if the bomb had gone off somewhere else along the bus's route.

The Afghans' need for healthcare was endless. Most of the Afghan refugees living in Pakistan had been there for a year or two, living in camps. There were shelter problems, their houses were built out of mud and straw. There were food problems, as there were few organizations distributing food then. While many of the Afghans had jobs, most were making just enough money to feed their families.

Our compound was directly across the street from Nasir Bagh, a large refugee camp. The lack of shelter, food, and clean water created a myriad of health issues: malnutrition, upper respiratory tract infections, skin diseases, diarrhea, malaria. These issues were far different from the ones I had treated in the United States, so I had to educate myself on infectious diseases, malnutrition, and other conditions so that I could teach the students. As refugees came to our clinic seeking care, the students received on-the-job training, preparing them for their return to Afghanistan.

The physical ailments were paired with psychosocial pain, as many Afghans had lost their loved ones and their livelihoods in the war. They all had a story to tell, how they lost daughters, brothers, mothers, sons. You could not help but feel some of their pain, share a small piece of their grief with them. I once met an older man who was having problems urinating. I asked him when he started to have trouble. "After I had to witness my sons being killed," he said.

We knew there were many more in need just across the border, but we were not allowed to operate inside Afghanistan because we could be captured or might be seen as spies. It was horrible not to be able to help. I would look off into the west at the end of the day and just think what it would be like to be over the hump of mountains that divided Pakistan and Afghanistan.

After about a month in Pakistan, my worldview had shifted beyond my life at home. I didn't think about my pension plan, my mortgage, my work, my car insurance. I started dreaming differently. My dreams were no longer centered on my family. My thoughts and energy were now consumed by how I could produce qualified medics who could cross the border and save the lives of people who were out of my reach, over a row of mountains that I could not cross.

After three months, I left Pakistan. Things in Hawaii did not feel the same. Few people were interested in what was happening in Afghanistan. Even fewer could relate to my experience there. I read everything I could get my hands on about Afghanistan and stayed on top of medical developments in communicable diseases, malnutrition, and other health issues in the developing world. I had caught a bug that I couldn't shake. What was supposed to be a one-time thing, the trip of a lifetime, had changed my life.

When, four years later, IMC called and asked me if I wanted to go back for another training program, I couldn't refuse. The first program had focused on trauma, wound care, and surgery, but this one would cover what the first one had missed, things like malnutrition, immunizations, mother-child care, infectious diseases, and land mine awareness.

When the Afghan medics came back to Pakistan for more supplies, we found that it was not wounds and injuries that were most common, but public health issues. As before, I was in Pakistan for three months. I felt revived, reconnected to the work I love.

I did not have my chance to go to Afghanistan until many years later. In February 2001, my wife died, and

I went through a terrible depression, plunging into what seemed like an abyss of grief, one I would never find the surface of. I was suicidal, indifferent to whether I lived or died.

Seven months later, 9/11 happened. I was on a fishing trip in Idaho with my brother and sons when I watched the second plane fly into the twin towers of the World Trade building on TV. I knew in that instant what I was going to do. I turned to my kids and said, "I am going to Afghanistan."

Everyone I knew thought I was crazy, but it was time to regain meaning in my life. I called IMC and told them that I was prepared to go if they needed me. I left shortly after.

When I arrived in Afghanistan, I realized how bad the conditions were. The need was unbelievable; everything was destroyed. Hospitals in Kabul were bursting at the seams, while the surrounding provinces had one clinic for every 50 thousand people. We worked around the clock, building 20 clinics in six weeks.

When our expatriate team arrived in Afghanistan, none of the modern world existed. There were no hair salons, no kite flying, no music. We could feel the flat affect of the Taliban on the people, on the streets, but slowly, as time went on, you would see one boy with a kite, then two. Every day there were more kites in the air. We started to hear music pour out of the homes onto the streets. It was thrilling to witness such a symbolic change, a hint of Afghanistan's potential after it was freed from the Soviet invasion and the Taliban.

Afghanistan saved me as I was working to save it. My life had found a renewed sense of purpose after the loss of my wife. It helped me surface from a deep despair that I thought I might never come out of. After years of wanting to cross the border, I was finally able to directly touch lives on the other side of those mountains that had tormented me during my first two missions in Pakistan.

After Afghanistan, I followed many more emergency response missions with IMC. I traveled with them to Liberia, Darfur, Indonesia, Iraq, Lebanon, and most recently, Kenya following the postelection violence.

When the tsunami shocked Southeast Asia, I sailed down the coast of Sumatra, Indonesia, in a leaking boat to find a place where foreign aid had not yet reached. I posed as a ship doctor on a cruise liner that was sent to evacuate foreigners so I could get into Lebanon when the country sealed its borders. I crossed into Iraq in an IMC convoy just 17 days after the bombing of Baghdad.

All these crises were different, yet there are always similarities. I learned what to look out for and how to make sure people get the care they need.

Each time I return home, I struggle to convey to friends and colleagues my experiences in the field. There are so many things we take for granted, like electricity, clean water, personal security, but there are millions around the world who get by without any of this. They pick themselves up and continue their lives even after they've lost everything. It was through these missions and the people I met on them that I found my own inner strength and resilience and the inspiration to move forward and discover deep fulfillment in loss. There is an Afghan proverb that says, "There is a way from heart to heart." There certainly was for me.

How Did I Get Myself into This?

~

LeAnn Thieman, LPN

ONE HUNDRED LITTLE babies lay three and four in a cardboard box, strapped in the belly of a gutted C130 cargo jet. Bombs exploded just miles away as we raced through 100-degree heat to save as many babies as possible. It was 1975 and Saigon was about to fall to the Communists.

With the first load of orphans on board, the American captain instructed us to prepare for takeoff. I wondered how you prepare 100 infants for this. Twenty-two cardboard boxes formed a row in the middle of the plane, and a long strap stretched from one end to the other, securing the boxes in place—a whole new definition of "seat belt safety." The sound of the motor was nearly deafening as the plane taxied down the runway. Its rumbling motion lulled the infants to near silence. We nine adults sat statuelike. Only the engine's roar broke the haunting, threatening stillness.

Finally the captain spoke. "We're out of range of the Vietcong. We're safe. We're going home!"

Whoops of gladness and relief filled the plane. Immediately, we volunteers unfastened our seat belts and hastened to tend to our charges.

Several large metal trash cans at each end of the row held food, formula, and other supplies. The commotion of loading babies hadn't allowed for feeding time; now all 100 of them were awake and crying simultaneously. In a frantic effort to rehydrate as many as we could as fast as we could, we propped bottles on the shoulders of each baby's squalling boxmate. As the bottles emptied, I flung a diaper over my shoulder and burped one baby at a time with my right hand, while bottle-feeding another with my left. My pediatric nurse experience prepared me for the infants' responses to stress, and soon the stuffy cargo compartment smelled of diarrhea and spit-up. The wee ones had started out so neatly dressed in homecoming outfits that were now wrinkled and soiled. We volunteers were disheveled, too, but there was merriment about it all. It was joyful work escorting babies to freedom, to families.

With one in my arms and two in my lap, I shook my head in disbelief and shouted above the cacophony:

"How did a mom and nurse get caught up in Operation Babylift?"

Ever since I was a little girl, I'd been drawn to the needs of orphans. At the annual church Thanksgiving clothing drives, a poster of a starving child hung on the podium: big, bloated belly; big, sad eyes filled with tears. It tugged at my heart. So my seven brothers and sisters and I went home and tried on all our hand-me-down clothes. If something didn't fit Bob, Denny, Roger, Diane, Mary, Theresa, or Keith, I tried it on since I was the runt of the litter. And if it didn't fit LeAnn, it went into the box for the poor. In retrospect, I think we were rather poor Iowa farm folk, but I felt rich when I could give that way.

We went trick-or-treating for UNICEF every Halloween. Our teachers gathered the whole school in the gymnasium, kindergartners through 12th graders—nearly 200 of us—and showed us film clips of Danny Kaye interacting with starving kids. Danny taught me that two and a half cents could buy a carton of milk and save a child's life. That's the first time in my life I began to believe we *are* our brother's keeper. We haven't been given everything we have in our lives to hoard, but to share.

I was still a little kid myself when I made a very important decision in my life, so important that I shared it on a special day. I was only 20 when Mark and I took our romantic walk along the creek and he asked me to marry him. No sooner had I said "yes!" than I told him about my dream to adopt a child someday. And from that day forward, it became *our* dream.

Maybe it was all these things that made me stop at a bake-sale booth as I strolled the mall in Iowa City in the early 1970s. I stared into the eyes of yet another starving poster child: big, bloated belly; big, sad eyes filled with tears. I wanted to help, to make a difference, so I picked up some cupcakes, some cookies, some bread, and a brochure and learned there was a meeting the next week. Hoping I could make a simple contribution, I attended and met a half-dozen young moms sitting around a chrome kitchen table with a dozen little kids running around. I learned about the cause, the needs of the orphans, and I signed on.

But my simple contribution got carried away when, in a few months, the chapter president moved away and I took on that role. Our home became the Iowa Chapter Headquarters of Friends of Children of Vietnam. This handful of women put drop boxes in grocery stores, went to doctors' offices for medications, hosted baby showers for orphans, and coordinated lots more bake sales. We raised over five tons of supplies and sent them to Vietnam in just three years.

I was completely blown away when the national headquarters called in April 1975 asking me to be the next escort to bring six—key word here, *six*—babies to their adoptive homes in the United States.

I had 24 hours to decide whether to go to Vietnam.

The decision was grueling. Could I leave my husband and two little girls to fly into a war zone? Calls to the U.S. State Department were reassuring. They promised the war was far from Saigon and was not predicted to escalate. We would be safe. Mostly I considered that Mark and I had applied to adopt a son through this same organization. Though we were on a two-year waiting list, I thought that my seeing his homeland would mean something to him someday.

After much thought and prayer, I agreed to go.

But between the time I said yes and the time I arrived, bombs began falling outside Saigon, President Ford had okayed Operation Babylift, and I arrived at the orphanage center in Vietnam to help rescue not 6, but 100 babies! Scores of infants covered every inch of floor in our two-story orphanage center. And in the midst of this chaos, a baby boy crawled into my arms, my heart, and our family. Our son had chosen us!

Now all 100 babies in a mammoth C-5 cargo jet were crying simultaneously. We propped countless bottles to feed the little ones. Some sucked the formula down in minutes, while others needed help. I cradled a baby girl in my crossed legs and coaxed her to drink with one arm, using my other hand to feed another baby. The nipple fell from the mouth of the one in my lap. Clearly she was too weak to suckle. Using both hands, I milked formula from the nipple to her mouth. While other babies protested, I continued until an ounce was taken. As the bottles emptied, we draped diapers over our shoulders and burped two at a time.

With one in my arms and two in my lap, I held and fed three infants at a time. Then I noticed a baby girl with a cleft palate, crying so hard she was hoarse. I picked up the wee one, and she rested limply in my lap. It didn't take a pediatric nurse to diagnose exhaustion and dehydration. Drop by drop, I squeezed formula from the bottle through her deformed lip.

The engine roared, the babies wailed, the walls vibrated, my heart ached as I listened to 99 babies protest while I gave undivided attention to one. Though it was difficult work, a sense of merriment danced among the volunteers—we were taking children to freedom, to families.

And I had a son.

Mercy Medical Center
Cedar Rapids Flood

∾

Chad Ware, RN

I AWOKE THE MORNING of June 12, 2008, knowing that the day was going to be one I would never forget. It was. I just never anticipated the magnitude to which that would come true. Throughout the week, the Cedar River, which runs right through the heart of Cedar Rapids, Iowa, had been rising. Record flooding in the city was anticipated. Evacuations of some neighborhoods had begun. On June 11, we opened our Incident Command Center at Mercy Medical Center.

My wife, Kate, was back home with her parents in Early, Iowa, dealing with her own crisis. Her mother had terminal cancer, and it had been decided that she should be moved into a nursing home. I was at home with two of our three girls, eight-year-old Emma and four-year-old Elise. Six-year-old Ellie was with her mom.

I have been involved in Disaster Preparedness at our hospital since 2001 and am part of a Federal Disaster Medical Assistance Team. I responded to Hurricanes Katrina, Rita, and Ike and was part of a Health and Human Services Mission in New Orleans. More than once I have left home on a moment's notice. Planning for a disaster has always been part of our family life. I just never expected my training to be put to use the way it was this time.

I awoke on June 12 to ongoing news reports of the flood. I listened to determine the safest exits off I-380, the main interstate through Cedar Rapids, and the only open bridge across the Cedar River.

I loaded up the girls and headed to the babysitter's house. When I dropped them off, I gave hugs and kisses. The sitter offered assurances that they would be safe and secure. I felt blessed to live in the community we do.

I continued on to work, only to find traffic backed up several miles on the interstate. When I finally got to the exit I needed, I found another line of traffic that was backed up. Once at the bottom of the ramp, I found out why: there was well over a foot of water flowing across the road.

I called my boss in the Emergency Department to check in and was told the hospital was on backup generator power but all our services were fully functioning. All our staff had made it in to work, and we were having an average morning in the Emergency Department.

I found deeper water in my path as I got closer to the hospital. A van had stalled in the roadway and the passengers had walked to the side of the road, safely out of the water. I followed the truck in front of me and kept progressing to the hospital. A truck coming from the other direction splashed a wave of water in front of it that eventually broke over the hood of my small SUV. I remembered my first sergeant from the military yelling at me as we were doing the same thing through a creek bed. "Don't take your foot off the gas," he would shout. I didn't and came out the other side. It took me another 15 minutes to traverse through the closed roads and one-way streets and travel the remaining three miles to the hospital.

I arrived to find the management team in the emergency room hard at work. Our electronic medical record system was functioning without a glitch. We began planning for an influx of patients.

Emergency Management is one of the programs I oversee for the department. Our Emergency Operations Center in the hospital was fully operational, and I ventured over there to see how things were going. Our focus had been on planning for an influx of patients from various sources, including other hospitals, as well as for the loss of power and steam.

River gauges were not working, and we had no accurate prediction of the amount of water coming our way.

The initial prediction was 24 to 26 feet, which would put the water at our doorstep. We were not anticipating the nearly 32 feet that came our way.

Throughout the day, we stayed in contact with our local Emergency Medical Service. They kept us informed, as did our Incident Command Center, regarding road closures and water levels.

Early in the afternoon, as the water continued to rise, we faced the realization that we might have to evacuate. I went upstairs to scout out an alternate patient care area to move the Emergency Department to. We had done this in previous years while working on evacuation plans, so I had a good idea of where to go. An eye surgery center on the first floor was a good option. The facility had been on backup power, so they had canceled all their cases for the day.

I started there and the staff showed me around and helped look at the possibilities. They were an incredible help. I went back to the department and talked with my director, Tami Meier. She and I worked out a plan in case we had to evacuate.

Once we thought we had a plan in place, we went back downstairs and talked to the staff. Most of our equipment, including cardiac monitors, exam equipment, and supply carts, was portable. Our documentation was on tablets, so as long as we had the wireless infrastructure, we were able to keep using our electronic medical record. We pulled out our paper templates just in case.

As the day went on, our toilets began to back up, as water from the city sewer system had nowhere else to go. Volunteers and hospital staff were sandbagging all around the south side of the building. The ambulance garage had a couple feet of water in it, and there was a very narrow path leading to the Emergency Department entrance that was dry.

I was helping one patient over the sandbags as another one was coming in with his mother. She was wearing an equalizer boot, a soft, pneumatic brace that accommodates the swelling patterns that occur throughout the rehabilitative process, and we had no way of easily assisting her over the pile of sandbags, which had grown to three feet in height. At that point, I realized we needed to move to higher ground.

Tami stayed downstairs to coordinate the move of the department. I went upstairs to prepare. The Emergency Department had 16 patients at the time. One was an acute stroke getting TPA, a drug used sometimes during a stroke or heart attack, to break up the clot that is causing the blockage. He was in a safe area of the department and elected to stay. We finished giving the medication and took the patient directly to the Intensive Care Center (ICC).

We had amazing support during that time. Staff and volunteers came from a number of different departments to help us move patients and equipment. Our local Emergency Medical System service was evacuating their dispatch area at the same time. They had to relocate all 911 equipment, radios, and office equipment. Even so, they helped coordinate communications regarding our move to a secondary location and, in the process, never dropped a 911 call!

Our Information Services Department was able to pull and reinstall wireless access points in less than an hour. That allowed us to maintain our wireless documentation system, so we were able to keep using our electronic medical records. Our patients remained incredibly calm throughout the process, and the patient care staff response to the rapidly changing situation was remarkable.

The evacuation of the Emergency Department went amazingly smoothly—in under an hour—and there were no status changes noted in any of our patients. Shortly after we evacuated, water started encroaching on our lab, radiology department, cath labs, ultrasound department, as well as into the basement where our pharmacy, central sterile room, and storeroom are located. All those departments were also directed to evacuate. Our staff members moved quickly and methodically, removing equipment, supplies, and medications from the basement and lower levels to higher ground.

Shortly after the evacuation of the Emergency Department, we lost all our diagnostic areas. The department leadership team, including our medical director, gathered to discuss whether we could continue to take patients. Without lab, radiology, or pharmacy, we could no longer diagnose and treat them.

There was another functioning Emergency Department within a half mile. The team went to the

Incident Command Center and discussed this with the command staff. Mercy leadership had come to the same conclusion and, at that point, the Emergency Department began diverting patients.

We continued to care for the patients we had admitted, or discharged them. Those who continued to come in were transferred to nearby St. Luke's Hospital. Tami Meier went back to the Emergency Department, now located on the first floor, to manage operations there. I was asked to stay within the Incident Command Center to help plan for the possibility of evacuating the entire hospital. Our chief medical officer, Dr. Mark Valliere, and I were assigned the task of working with the directors and managers of the inpatient floors to plan the details of our hospitalwide evacuation.

Our plan called for a reverse triage process, meaning the least ill patients would be evacuated first. We called the group together and explained the possibility of having to evacuate. Nurses were directed to assess their patients, determine transport needs, and notify family members. Physicians came in to help triage patients and discharged those capable of going home. Fortunately, there were a number of discharges planned for the next morning. During this meeting, in consultation with our Intensive Care Center medical director, it was decided that it would be best to evacuate our six ICC patients and three Neonatal Intensive Care Unit (NICU) patients while we still had backup power and nearby St. Luke's had beds to accept them. The evacuation of those patients began at approximately 8:00 P.M.

The decision to evacuate the entire hospital came a short time later. Dr Valliere coordinated with the State Public Health Department to locate beds and arrange transport. The complete evacuation began after midnight.

We decided to divert from the reverse triage process, as we still had power to the elevator. We wanted to get our most difficult patients transferred first, while we still had functioning elevators. The ICC and NICU had already been evacuated, so we moved to the next unit with the most acutely ill patients: the Cardiac Stroke Center. As ambulances arrived, we coordinated bringing patients down to the only hospital entrance untouched by floodwater. We used VHF radios to coordinate patient transfers with ambulance arrivals.

Our staff set up a checkpoint at the exit to ensure accountability. We kept a log identifying the patients, where they were going, what ambulance was taking them, what time they left, and when they arrived at the receiving facility. As patients boarded outgoing ambulances, vans, or buses, Mercy staff checked to make sure they all had a hard copy of their medical records with them.

Shortly after we had started the evacuation, I remember our president and CEO, Tim Charles, coming up behind me and saying, "Chad, we have a problem." I remember thinking, *What other problem could there be?!* He was so calm and confident. He explained that water was coming into the building in key areas that could affect power to the elevators. His thoughtful leadership and that of our administration were certainly key to our success during this crisis. They stayed calm and supportive. We stayed calm and got the job done.

The uncertainty about our power supply hastened our efforts to begin at the ninth floor of our patient tower to bring all patients down. Directors and nurse managers went back to their floors to coordinate the process.

One of the physicians who had come in to assist had previously been a paramedic and had experience in staging ambulances. He went out and began staging all our transport vehicles. We needed someone to coordinate the floor-to-floor evacuation; another one of our physicians secured a radio and took care of it.

I moved our checkpoint and bed assignment area closer to the exit. Communication with the State Public Health Department was maintained, and it continued to identify available beds throughout the state for our patients. Our social workers worked with our Hallmar staff (a 55-bed long-term care facility within the hospital) to arrange for beds within local care centers in the community. By 8:00 A.M. the next morning, we had evacuated all 183 patients.

I look back in awe. Our patient care staff was amazing. They kept patients calm and informed. I remember walking up and down the line of patients as they waited to be transferred. They smiled, laughed, and even made a few jokes. Keeping our patients safe was our primary goal. The nurses loaded patients into ambulances, then sat in the congested hallways on cell phones with flashlights, calling reports to the receiving hospitals. Nurses volunteered for round-trip transports, some as long as six hours, to ensure our patients were supported during the evacuation.

I must also mention our maintenance staff, volunteers, and construction contractors who were down on the ground and basement floors, sandbagging and pumping water from the building to protect our electrical systems. At times, many stood in five feet of water on the south perimeter of the building. Those people are also unsung heroes of this disaster.

I cannot say enough about the way everyone on our staff came together. Our patient care staff not only took care of patients but sometimes stacked sandbags or helped push water toward pumps.

The response we had from the community was amazing. Hundreds of people showed up to assist us. In the weeks leading up to the flood, we had major construction projects going on within the hospital, including the Emergency Department. The construction contractors showed up with their crews and worked side by side with our Maintenance Department, fixing electrical and plumbing, sandbagging, and pumping out water. I don't think I've ever felt so proud to be a part of any organization or community as I did on that Friday the 13th!

Our marketing department developed an advertisement campaign to thank the community. They used the most inspirational picture I've ever seen. It showed a line of volunteers, hospital staff, and construction workers under the night lights of the ED in waist-high water, sandbagging.

There are many amazing stories of selfless acts throughout this event. One was when our Maintenance Department cut a template out of plywood to push back water coming through a two-foot-wide vent pipe and then bolted it in place. This kept water out of key electrical panels. Another was when one of our contractors, who knew the facility very well, called from another state and directed one of the electricians to a key electrical panel through a winding basement corridor, in the dark. Another was when a nurse who, when no one else from that floor was available, volunteered to take a six-hour trip in a wheelchair van transport to ensure a patient got the proper medications. And a cardiologist came from his office in scrubs and a lab coat and jumped in to help with sandbagging efforts.

Above all, as I look back on this disaster, I can truly say we put our patients first. The hospital evacuated 183 patients with no decline in patient status and no deaths. In addition, despite the odds, on Monday, just three days later, we were able to begin serving patients once again. Within 15 days, all hospital services were operational.

Ground Zero:
A Paramedic's Perspective

~

Sandra (Sam) Bradley, EMT-P

I STILL HAVE THE program from Christian's funeral. The cover picture shows his last name, Regenhard, written on his helmet in black marker across gray duct tape. He was 28 years old and had graduated from the Fire Academy only six weeks before 9/11. He died on September 11, 2001. I wish I had known him.

I came from California, along with the other members of my federal Disaster Medical Assistance Team, and stood in the street in uniform along with firefighters from Las Vegas, Seattle, and Vancouver. I had taken part in quite a number of firefighter funerals in my 22 years as a paramedic, but never experienced anything like this. St. Patrick's Cathedral, circa 1879, loomed large in front of us, sitting majestically in the middle of midtown Manhattan. It was awe-inspiring. It was also incongruous with the Fifth Avenue shops in near proximity, like Versace and Cartier. The church was open; the stores were closed. Who knew when fashion would regain any level of importance in New York City? Who knew when New York would once again be New York?

The sad whine of the bagpipes and the steady rhythm of the snare drum started the procession. We stood at attention as a fire engine, draped in black cloth, moved slowly up Fifth Avenue toward the church. It was followed by dozens of solemn firefighters in Class A uniform, and black limousines that carried the grieving family.

When the team had decided to go to at least one memorial, we had a large schedule of them to choose from. We picked this one because it was early enough in the morning for us to attend, giving us enough time before our afternoon shift at Ground Zero. We all felt strongly that we wanted to do this as a team. The numbers of memorials were overwhelming, and we had never met any of these firefighters, but our feeling was that if we could honor one, we could honor them all.

There were three thousand people at Christian's memorial. I was proud to be one of them. The ceremony combined Catholic Liturgy and ceremonies of honor by the Fire Department of New York City and the U.S. Marines. By the time the flags were lowered and we walked away, we felt we had known him.

In the next few days, after a phone call to his mother, we were invited to a private showing of Christian's artwork in Brooklyn. We met his family and learned more about this talented young man and his connections to San Francisco through his art and his family stories. We decided to make him an honorary team member. We gave his mother a team T-shirt and a patch. She gave us some things of Christian's.

On September 11, 2001, I was coming on duty for my 24-hour shift as an ambulance company paramedic supervisor. I hadn't listened to the radio in the car that morning. The tense, bewildered expression on the departing supervisor's face as he stared in the window of my SUV was my first clue that this wasn't going to be a normal shift.

Dave took me into the classroom of our California office where we normally conduct safety and EMT classes. The room has a large television and is a common gathering place for the employees. I watched with a roomful of stunned emergency medical technicians and paramedics as the first tower fell. It was surreal. I knew then that it was going to be a long and bizarre 24 hours. We had to figure out how all this was going to affect us and wondered if there would be more terrorist acts to come.

Shortly thereafter, there was a fatal traffic collision in the far east part of our county. The fire department called for a medical helicopter. Moments later I received the call from the helicopter service, advising us they had just been grounded. It was the first ripple effect we felt all the way on the West Coast.

The next evening, I went to teach my emergency medical technician class at the local community college. We were only about one month into the semester. Student ages ran from 18 to 25 years, with a smattering of older folks. They all wore the same stunned expression that day. I wondered what the impact would be on them, these predominantly young people with aspirations of becoming firefighters. In our world of emergency medical services people, firefighters and cops were all part of a large extended family. If one was killed in the line of duty, the loss was felt by all of us as keenly as if they were blood relations. Three hundred and forty-three were lost in one day in New York City. We were only beginning to feel the true impact of that as numbness and disbelief turned to reality and fear. The students stared at me like deer in headlights as I stood at the front of the room. They expected me to explain it to them. They wanted me to make it all right. I let them talk and wondered how many of them would continue on their current career path and how many would seek a safer vocation.

A 16-member contingent of doctors, nurses, mid-level practitioners, EMTs, paramedics, and a pharmacist were chosen from our team in California to work in concert with two similar teams from other states. Our mission was to provide care to the firefighters, heavy equipment workers, police, and other recovery workers inside the secure perimeter of Ground Zero.

Our Liberty treatment site offered us a view of the "pile," and we watched as the ironworkers painstakingly tore down what was left of the metal structures bit by bit. Our Church Street treatment site backed up against a church cemetery. If you were to look out the back doors, you would be greeted with the disconcerting sight of headstones covered in dirt and ash. Looking up into the trees, you would see swatches of colored cloth hanging from the branches, clothing that had been worn by the people who perished there.

The site workers came to us with lacerations and burns. The firefighters needed us but feared that we would take them away from the work they were obsessed with: finding their lost brethren. When they did come, they were hardly able to breathe. We'd give them a treatment and send them off again, praying for their physical and mental health. We knew it was too late for many.

The air was thick and we had to wear double-filter respirators when we went outside. The noise of heavy earth-moving equipment was constant. The only time the noise stopped was when three horns were sounded. We all knew what that meant: another body was found. One day we watched the ritual no fewer than 30 times: stop the equipment, back in the ambulance, drape a flag over the body, and place it in the ambulance. Six firefighters would then throw down their tools and walk alongside the ambulance as it exited the pile. Every time, there was a heavy silence. Every time, there was reverence. Every time, my heart broke, although I comforted myself with the thought that another family would have closure.

As we were ending our shift that same night, one of the firefighters I had talked with several times came by our Church Street tent and told me, "You have to go by the Ten House—there's something happening there." The Ten House had been where Engine Ten and Ladder Ten had been stationed on the periphery of the towers. They were the first-due companies on September 11. They lost six firefighters that day. The station had been damaged but was still standing and had become a place of solace and refuge for those working Ground Zero.

A crane was moving a huge metal statue of a firefighter from the bed of a small pickup when we arrived there. As the story goes, a woman in Seattle had been commissioned to build a statue of a firefighter with a pike pole in his hands. When the towers went down, she asked if she could donate it to New York City. She replaced the pike pole with a flag and drove it across the country. As it hit the ground, all the stress of the day welled up in me and the floodgates opened. I wasn't ashamed and I wasn't alone. Firefighters, filthy from their day's work, watched with appreciation. They were just as taken with this as I was. This act of kindness was just what we needed to defuse a long day of sick firefighters, damaged ironworkers, and a multitude of body recoveries.

It was after midnight when our bus would drop us off at our hotel in Times Square. Most of us were still fired up and wanted to hear what the other half of the team had experienced that day. A restaurant across the street looked forward to seeing us. New Yorkers weren't going out much. They were still hunkered down and licking their wounds. The only customers the restaurant had besides us were the firefighters coming in from all over the world to pay their respects at the multitude of memorial services. As soon as we arrived, plates of hot french fries were brought to our table. We'd wash them down with martinis, arguing about whether vodka or gin was better and whether there should be two or three olives. The running joke was, "Let's have just one." It never was.

Everything I'd heard about New York was different from what I experienced. The infamous sound of honking horns in the streets of Times Square was absent. There was no rudeness from the workers in the deli where we got our lunch, and no one tried to run us over if we jaywalked. On the contrary, people would stop us on the street and ask us if we were "out there." They couldn't thank us enough for coming to help their broken city after they found out we'd come all the way from California.

A few days before we left, I was working the Liberty tent with my friend, Andy, an RN. This night was unique because it was the first time the constant drone of heavy equipment had stopped. The first public showing of the site would be the next morning. A pastor came in several times asking for eyewash. Our Commander, Dave, asked what was going on. It seems the firefighters were taking advantage of the moment to dig into an area where they had been trying to look for remains. It was an old-fashioned bucket brigade. Dirt from the unstable ceiling was falling into their eyes. Dave looked at Andy and me and said, "Get your gear; you're going up there." Andy and I looked at each other. Up there?

Minutes later we were dropped off with our advanced life support gear. The idea was for us to be available if any of the firefighters were injured or, God forbid, the ceiling caved in on them. We found ourselves looking down into a very large hole. The captain in charge saw us and waved us down. He wanted us to go down there.

Andy and I were standing in the middle of the deepest part of the most infamous place in the world. We looked at each other, but with respirators covering our faces we could only speak with our eyes. We saw pieces of rebar, ribbed poles of steel used to reinforce concrete structures from Tower Two sticking out of the ground; papers blown out of tower windows just before their recipients followed them; and a parking ticket that lay at my feet. The air was thick with dirt, smoke, and ash. We could feel the heat in our steel-toed boots as the underground area below us still burned, fed by the jet fuel. Andy and I have only ever spoken of this lightly, even to this day, but we both had the distinct feeling that we were not alone. It was the eeriest sensation I've ever experienced. I remember, as an ER tech, when I had to wrap a recently deceased body that I sometimes felt the presence of the departing spirit. I always said good-bye. I said good-bye that day to several thousand people. I prayed that they could find peace.

As they wrapped up the unsuccessful operation, the firefighters walked quietly up the path to the top of the hole where we had been. For whatever reason, they stood in a line along the perimeter of the hole, looking down. Andy and I were looking. I'm sure they were thinking about the bodies they hadn't found and the knowledge that this had probably been their last chance to find them. The sadness was pervasive. They were shrouded in the thick, almost opaque air. There was a huge bank of lights behind them that gave them an almost supernatural backlight. Andy and I looked at each other and knew this vision would be forever burned into our minds along with understanding of the mind-numbing fatigue, helplessness, and despair that they were feeling. In a matter of days, the city would be pulling the plug on the recovery operation. They were coming to terms with the fact that most of the remains would never be recovered.

Assimilation back into what were supposed to be our normal lives took weeks, at least to the extent that our lives were ever to be "normal" again. Coming home to hearing about broken dishwashers, unruly kids, and piled-up bills didn't break through our apathy for the mundane. Sitting through meaningless business meetings was aggravating and painful. Our concept of "bad" and "evil" had taken on a whole new meaning. Our brains were still wrapped up with families that would never have closure on their loved ones and firefighters who were destined to be physically devastated and psychologically impaired. We consider ourselves lifesavers, but there was nothing we could do for these people but put salve on their burns, bandages on their lacerations, and clear their lungs temporarily. I can only hope that the short interactions we had with them mattered and gave them something positive.

Most of our Ground Zero contingents are still with the team. Andy and I work in the same EMS system and see each other regularly. We bonded in a way that no one else could ever understand. Some of the team members are still in touch with Christian's family. Many of us wrote articles and did public speaking on the experience. Everyone wanted to know what it was like "out there." Others went on to work at the Katrina hurricane disaster in 2005, which, in some respects, made the World Trade Center experience seem like a walk in the park. Some of us have lingering psychological trauma. Despite that, we are grateful and honored to have served our country and the people of New York City. None of us will ever forget.

Sleepless in the Sahara

~

Louise M. Robinson, RN

AFTER THE CEASE-FIRE was declared in the Persian Gulf War, a refugee camp was discovered not far from the southern border of Iraq. When the war closed off the borders of Iraq and Kuwait, the people caught in the middle of the desert had nowhere to go: Turks, Bedouins, Iranians, Kuwaitis, Iraqis, Saudi Arabians. The camp grew as people gathered together for safety.

The International Red Cross took over management of the camp and contacted Red Cross headquarters in Washington, D.C. The call went out for volunteers. As an International Red Cross volunteer disaster nurse, I answered that call. Our mission was to be called Operation Desert Care.

Red Cross representatives met 14 of us medical volunteers at the airport in Saudi Arabia, and we rode in a three-car convoy for five hours to the Kuwait border. Even in the darkness, we could feel the isolation of the desert as we bumped over and around bomb craters in the road. After reaching the border, we drove on another hour to a bombed-out airport. From there we were escorted to Kuwait City's Sahara Hotel, our home for the next three months.

The entire hotel had been leased for the use of the International Red Cross League. Sometimes it had electricity, sometimes water. Rarely both. The hotel was slowly recovering from the ravages of the war. It was as clean as possible in those circumstances.

The next morning we headed out for the refugee camp. We drove up the "Alley of Death," horrible enough on television back home, but unspeakable in real life: bomb craters, burned-out military and civilian vehicles, some with skeletal remains still inside.

We drove past the oil well fires, through the foul-smelling blackness, and out the other side. Eyes burning, we coughed as we continued up the road to the refugee camp. At the camp, we assessed the needs of the people with regard to sanitation, water, and food.

About seven thousand people had already divided themselves into sections according to nationality, with bachelors and families in separate areas. I was assigned the Iraqi area and given an excellent interpreter, who lived in the camp with his family. Educated in Europe as a civil engineer, Asad spoke four languages.

The camp was surrounded by mines that hadn't been cleared by the military. Every once in a while, we heard a big "whump!" as a mine exploded when a camel or a person—usually a child—stepped on it. The refugees were provided with small stoves and fuel, but some preferred cooking fires. When the children went out beyond the camp's perimeters to gather firewood, they might step on a hidden mine or find a pretty, shiny object that exploded when they picked it up, with horrible consequences.

On our first day at the camp someone yelled, "There's been a bomb! We need nurses!" We ran to the medical tent to find two seriously injured men. We started IVs and bandaged pieces together for the ambulance ride to the hospital in Kuwait City. Ten minutes later, we heard a call about a woman collapsing. Out we went again.

Then we set up social service tents and separate medical tents for men and women. We established guidelines for the distribution of food and water and for trash pickup to lessen the chance of cholera and typhoid.

During the two-hour drive back to Kuwait City, we discussed what we had seen and what we could do to make things better for these unfortunate people. We all felt an adrenaline rush, but we were still overwhelmed. None of us had previous experience dealing with this level of disaster. We took that mind-numbing drive through the horrible Valley of Death, past the oil well fires like an image of Hell.

The Iraqis in my area were cooperative, organizing themselves into sections. One section leader challenged another to see who had the cleanest area. We attempted the same with the Bedouins, but it was an uphill battle. They were accustomed to wandering the desert. Anything they threw away, and it wasn't much, just disappeared into the vastness. The concept of trash pickup was difficult for them.

A wonderful toilet tent was set up in the administration section. It was just a hole in the ground, but it had all the amenities: toilet paper. The medical and pharmacy tents were shaping up as well. We were all filthy, hot, exhausted, and loving it.

Every afternoon we drove over two hours back to the hotel for showers, if there was water. At dinner we discussed what we had done that day and what we hoped to accomplish the next day.

Often I was sleepless in the Sahara Hotel. Images of the camp haunted me: the heat, the smoke, and the people torn away from their homes. The refugees were afraid Saddam's forces would come into the camp to kill them, and asked us to put barbed wire around the entire camp. This was a difficult concept for us Americans, too reminiscent of the concentration camps of World War II.

One of the ongoing problems was the arrival—or nonarrival—of water trucks. Three trucks had been hired to bring water to the camp three times a week. Sometimes they didn't come at all.

We set up a registration system for the people seen in the medical tent. Using their real names could be dangerous for some of them. We simply requested they use the same name whenever they came. The registration cards helped us keep track of what illnesses and injuries were prevalent and enabled us to follow up on the patients who needed to be seen again.

There was an ambulance at the camp for transporting seriously ill or injured people to the hospital in Kuwait City, but refugees could not return to Kuwait on their own.

Most of the camp supplies were donations, and we often had to wait for them. Sometimes they showed up, sometimes not. We had to make do with what we had. On occasion we got donations of different military Meals Ready to Eat (MREs), some American, some British, even once a French one that we fought over, then shared. One day we discovered all the toilet paper was gone from our lovely toilet tent, so we made do with various communications sent out from headquarters. Probably the best use for them.

One day, one of the Kuwaiti staff ran into the tent yelling that someone had been burned. The two-man tents that China had generously donated were extremely flammable, but some refugees insisted on cooking inside them. They brought in two men, one slightly singed, the other badly blistered on his hands, arms, and one leg. We got them taken care of without disturbing our volunteer doctor, who had been caring for patients nonstop for 36 hours. I was glad we didn't have to wake him.

Most mornings progressed with the usual struggle to obtain things we had been promising people for days. Finally, one day we were told the water truck had arrived and the bulldozer was there to dig the trash trenches, all at the same time. We were ecstatic! We organized the water truck setup and went off to show the bulldozer operator where to start. The refugees gathered around and had a great time arguing about how everything should be done.

The next day, I inspected the trash pits. They looked great! Some even had trash in them! They also had kids in them looking for anything interesting.

That same afternoon, I met with the Iraqi section leader, Mohammed, and his two section chiefs. Mohammed was very hospitable and invited us to meet in his tent, furnished with beautiful rugs and hangings. His wife served us tea in gold-rimmed cups. So lovely after our lunch of cold beans, eaten directly out of the can.

After a month or so, a United Nations contingent set up a tent in the camp to help relocate some of the refugees. These were ordinary people caught in the middle of a bad situation: engineers, doctors, merchants, shopkeepers, office workers. We discovered a lawyer and his family in the Kuwaiti section and their former servants in the Irani section. War is a great equalizer.

Some mornings the sky was black, visibility about 500 feet at best. The wind came from the direction of the oil well fires, and we had to drive slowly in case a car or camel suddenly appeared out of the smoke. It was always windy at the camp. I must have eaten more dust than had been under my bed in the last 20 years.

One day a 14-year-old girl whose family had all been killed in Iraq was brought into camp. One of our translators, Sindice, and her family kindly took her in. I am always touched by the generosity of people with little to share.

At the Sahara Hotel sometimes I woke up in the night to the sound of stray cats mating. Not a pleasant sound at three in the morning, but preferable to gunfire. I thought I would get used to the sound of gunfire, but I still woke with my heart pounding. Usually, though, it was nightmares that woke me. I am still haunted by the image of the women and children waiting for water trucks that never came.

We got a day or two off every week. Sometimes I just slept all day, and sometimes a group of us went shopping. It was good to see the shops opening again in Kuwait City, and the people looking less frightened. One day we saw that a Hardees fast food place had reopened! We all had hot dogs and fries. While I was taking photos of the people and shops, a woman stopped us.

"You should have seen this city before, when it was beautiful!" she sobbed.

I reassured her that it would be beautiful again. We parted with the traditional *Inshallah*. God willing, her home would be beautiful again.

The last month at the camp was busy and heartening. The United Nations made arrangements for many refugees to be transported to other countries. One morning, as we drove into camp, we passed a huge truck loaded with refugees going to Iran. There was much excitement and waving good-bye.

It was a typical day in the camp. I walked over to the water truck delivery site and talked with the women waiting there. They requested soap and the removal of live ammo lying around the camp. A reasonable request. I checked my Iraqi area and clinic, then took a jacket to an albino Bedouin and gave him my hat and Chapstick. On a walk-through of my Iraqi area with my translator, Asad, we met an old woman who asked if we could help her get teeth. I had to tell her we couldn't. Then her family asked if we could get her a husband. We all enjoyed the joke as I pretended to add it to my list. Following my walk-through, I worked at the women's clinic doing triage. Everyone grinned and applauded when a healthy baby was born.

Our time was running out and the camp was winding down. More people left for Iran. By now there were only about a thousand people left on the Iraqi side, with nine hundred or so leaving soon for Iran or Saudi Arabia. Plenty of food came in, plenty of water, plenty of sand and wind.

Our toilet tent blew away, so no one peed all afternoon. We stopped at a U.S. Army base on the way back to the hotel to use their latrines. What luxury! Toilet paper and even seats!

Asad, my wonderful interpreter, invited me to have tea with his family. Asad's mother, a woman near my own age, had been killed in the first days of the war. At tea there were several giggling little kids, his nieces and nephews. They called giggling children "mosquitoes."

The sky was very overcast with smoke from the oil well fires. This kept the heat down, but I wondered what it was doing to our lungs.

We returned from camp exhausted, to find the electricity out in the hotel. No elevators, showers in the dark. It was 120 degrees the next day. We saw 148 people at the clinic.

Some refugees brought in an old woman covered in dust, her sandals tied on with rope. She said the Kuwaiti soldiers at the checkpoint took her identification cards and told her to come to the Red Cross camp to be taken care of while they checked her out. She told us her story: she had gone to Iraq to look for her son, who was in prison, although she was afraid he might have been killed. She looked for him in Iraq for two months, but never found him. Now this determined old woman was walking back to Kuwait—more than 300 miles!—to rejoin her family.

I got her food and water and found a family for her to stay with. Patrick, with the International Committee of the Red Cross, called her family in Kuwait to let them know she was here and arranged her transportation back home. She thanked us, cried a little, and fell asleep.

I walked the Iraqi side, talking to people, listening to their hopes and fears. Rumors floated around the camp that Saudi Arabia was willing to take some refugees. Some people were eager to go, but others feared they might be killed there. The Bedouins were asking how long they would have to stay in the camp. The desert was full of land mines. Where does a nomad go when you take away his desert?

Toward the end of my deployment, the work at the clinic became a little easier—no hidden mines blowing off hands or feet for a day, thank Allah.

On the last day at the camp, all the remaining Iraqis were ready to leave. Asad was upset. He wanted to stay and help me, but he had been told he must leave with his family. I went to his tent to say good-bye to him and his wonderful family. Asad gave me a beautiful Iraqi one-dinar coin so I would remember them. As if I could forget. He told me I had been like a mother to him since his own was gone. It was only then I learned he had also lost his wife and child at the beginning of the war. All the little mosquitoes waved and called "Goot pie, goot pie!" to me as I left.

There was no time for tears; we saw 167 patients in three hours. The generator for the clinic lights was not working, so we held flashlights for the doctor while he treated a man's injured foot and sutured a cut on a girl's face.

I spent the rest of the day with the United Nations dozers and the ordinance team. We found grenades and other weapons left behind by the Iraqis. They had been terribly afraid for their lives for a very long time. Long after the sun set, the buses came to take the remaining Iraqis to the airport. As I had promised, I was there to wave good-bye, to see the hope and optimism on the faces of these people who had come to mean so much to me.

Asad and his family were on the last bus, the children laughing and waving as they drove away.

"Goot pie, my little mosquitoes," I whispered. "May Allah watch over you."

Fronting Up to a Civil Emergency

~

Julie Vickery, RN, BN, PGCert

In february 2004, the lower North Island in Manawatu, New Zealand, suffered a period of very heavy rainfall, resulting in severe and extensive flooding. This civil emergency worsened over four days, leaving townships flooded, people evacuated from their homes, and limited power, water, sewerage, and communication. The worst-hit areas remained without services for weeks.

MidCentral District Health Board's (DHB) district nursing service covers a wide area, operating 24 hours a day. We have six bases covering the Horowhenua, Manawatu, Feilding, and Tararua regions, all of which were severely affected by the extreme weather and subsequent flooding. This is a story of the experience of maintaining services and caring for patients during the developing civil emergency.

It had been raining all weekend. I had hardly been outside, marooned in the house by unrelenting curtains of rain. By Sunday night I was thinking that things might be getting serious. So when I woke to the 6:30 A.M. news on Monday, February 16, to hear that the Oroua River had breached its banks, I wasn't that surprised, but I was worried and my thoughts raced. How extensive was the flooding? What areas were affected? Would we be able to see our patients? Did the night nurse get home safely? My rather bemused family watched me rush out the door to work.

I arrived at our Palmerston North Hospital base to find that the night nurse was running late. She had been to visit a patient near Sanson and had to take a long detour home, as a bridge had been washed out. She and her driver were safe, but very tired. It had been a long night, with travel to Dannevirke also disrupted by the heavy rain, requiring detours.

Staff members were phoning in to say they were unable to get to work. Some nurses were able to travel to other bases and help out there. My first act was to check the civil emergency policy. It began with the words: "The team leader will…" My team leader, Cushla Roache, was trapped in Feilding. I was going to have to get on with it myself!

During such large-scale events, the hospital establishes a central communication center to coordinate information and services in the hospital and wider community. I rang the number, but there was no dial tone. Oh, well, I reasoned, it was only 8:00 A.M.; they would barely be at work yet.

I contacted the risk management officer and explained I would need accurate information regarding road closures and alternative routes, as we had approximately 750 patients scattered across both urban and rural locations, some of whom had to be seen within four hours. He sounded rather shocked by the numbers, but I reassured him we wouldn't need to see them all at once! Cushla rang to say that she and one of the Feilding office nurses had been able to get to the central communications center, with the help of the police, and were contacting as many of the local patients as they could.

Water was lapping at the steps of the building, and much of the town was already underwater. They had identified the patients urgently needing attention, one of whom would need to be brought over to Palmerston North to ensure her intravenous therapy could be continued and her condition monitored. Many of these patients were being evacuated, and tracking them down would be a challenge over the next 24 hours. The team leader also gave some much needed moral support and advice. It was great having her on the spot, as transport in and out of the area was impossible.

Having checked in with all the bases, we saw clearly that Feilding was the worst affected. Access in and out of Palmerston North was limited, but all other areas were accessible locally. The nurses were trying to contact their patients to give them practical advice and reassurance that we would make our calls as soon as the roads were cleared.

By 9:00 A.M. I had assessed the immediate situation, identifying where the most urgent needs were. Information was finally coming through from the now established communication center. Accurate information regarding road closures and alternative routes enabled me to redeploy nurses within their local areas. For example, a nurse living in Shannon couldn't get to her usual workplace at Foxton, but she was able to help in Levin. A number of nurses were unable to leave their homes at all and found it incredibly frustrating not being able to use their skills to help others. There was a real sense of the team pulling together to make the best of the situation and think creatively about how to reach patients.

I kept in touch with as many of our nurses as I could to see where they would be of most value. Many stayed in their local areas and worked with the Civil Defence. Once our own patients were accounted for and contacted, these nurses' wealth of expertise was much needed.

I stayed in regular contact with the only nurse who was able to reach the Pahiatua Base, Marie Taplin. She had been able to see all her patients, except a man an hour away on a metal road. This man had phoned to say the road was passable, but after driving for 30 minutes and negotiating several small slips, she turned back, feeling very insecure in her small, lightweight vehicle. Marie told me she felt guilty that she had been unable to see this patient, but I reassured her that she had done the right thing and that, if necessary, we could use emergency services to get to him.

As the day wore on and the weather was showing no sign of letting up, we arranged for five of our acute hospital-in-the-home patients to be brought in from outlying areas and put up in motels in Palmerston North. These patients were all receiving IV therapy and needed close monitoring.

This proved to be a wise move, as the following day the situation became even worse. More roads were closed, and the coastal towns were now underwater and being evacuated. Phone contact was down in these areas, and I prepared to have two patients evacuated to Palmerston North. Fortunately, this was not necessary, but it was reassuring to have the coordination of emergency services.

The team in the communication center was a huge help. I only had to explain our requirements and they were able to coordinate all the outside help. Because of road closures, one of the Dannevirke district nurses, Sarah Wadley, came back to work at 11:00 P.M. for several nights to administer IV therapy to one of our patients.

The emergency continued for one further day in the Palmerston North region, but by Wednesday afternoon we were able to return our motel patients to their homes. One young man had come to support his brother. The pair thoroughly enjoyed the motel amenities and seemed a bit disappointed when we were able to get them home!

While many roads were still closed, we were able to get to most of our patients by this stage, albeit with long detours, greatly increasing travel time. This was particularly difficult for our night nurse and her care assistant, who were seeing patients across the wider region during the course of the night. By Thursday, four days into the storm, all but the worst-hit areas were able to get back to business as usual.

The following weeks were somewhat surreal. In Palmerston North all was normal, but within a 20-minute drive, there were people without homes or the basic necessities of clean water and power. Food supplies were disrupted and a huge cleanup was under way. Many of our nurses were torn between helping their families and friends and coming to work to care for patients.

I spoke with our referral nurse, Ros Meads, with whom I share an office. While I knew that Ros had to make big detours to get to work, and that her farm had suffered much damage, it wasn't until I sat and really listened to her that I began to understand what it meant to be a working nurse, wife, mother, friend, and member of a ravaged community, all at the same time. Coming to work was not only a physical effort; fulfilling all the other roles to support family and friends was creating dilemmas and stresses. Ros described the daily journey to work as eerie, like leaving another planet where farms were devastated and families were experiencing water and power outages, to arrive in Palmerston North where everything was back to normal.

By the end of the following week, the huge outpouring of energy and adrenaline needed to cope with the emergency had drained away, and staff and patients were left tired and irritable. The nurses who were still coping with the aftereffects of flood damage and limited power and water supplies were especially vulnerable, working with colleagues for whom it was business as usual.

One nurse told me of some of her patients' experiences. Two elderly patients were still living in a hotel four months later because their flat wouldn't be habitable for months. Another woman's leg ulcer had deteriorated badly because she was unable to be seen for 48 hours during the flooding. One gentleman was writing to his landlord to apologize for not giving sufficient notice of leaving his flat. He had been evacuated by emergency services at 2:00 A.M.!

In the aftermath were the personal and professional reviews. I took part in the District Health Board–wide formal debrief, where I was able to present our nursing perspective to the wider group. Within the service I arranged for nurses to have the opportunity to share stories and review the emergency procedure documents at team meetings. It was really valuable for me to hear these experiences and to add them to my own perspective. I was humbled by the ways our team had pulled together, supporting each other and going the extra mile to continue to provide the best care possible for our patients. MidCentral's district nursing service—all 75 of us—was a great team!

Bent but Not Broken

~

Linda Garrett, RN

I REMEMBER FROM CATHOLIC school that nuns can be very persuasive. Sister Ramona, a 74-year-old Franciscan nun from Harlingen, Texas, was no exception.

In the fall of 2005, after Hurricane Katrina, I worked on a mental health team with the American Red Cross in Gautier and Moss Point, Louisiana. I was assigned with Sister Ramona. What an amazing woman! She had been all over the world. Her sole mission in life was to do good and make the lives of other people better. She was a hoot to work with. A fixture at the base, she circulated and schmoozed so that she could get clothing donations to give away on our many runs out into the community.

I got in the car with Sister Ramona and threw my bag of dirty laundry in the backseat. As we drove, we received a panicked call from headquarters and were instructed to visit a man named Robert, who had been staying at a motel. He had terminal brain cancer and was not expected to live out the month, but every time someone tried to see him, he was not there.

We got him this time. Tall and emaciated, he said he was on 20 different meds, but the only one we saw was an antihistamine. "The rest is in my truck," he told us, but wouldn't tell us where the keys were so we could check them. He also told us he was diabetic, but we saw no supplies to indicate that.

Suddenly, he began cramping, doubled over, and appeared to be in extreme pain. I wanted to call an ambulance, but Robert said he'd refuse it. With the shortage of vehicles, manpower, and services post-Katrina, ambulance crews left immediately if the patient refused help.

Sister Ramona did her best, using her most persuasive techniques. Robert had told us he'd attended Catholic school when he was growing up in New Orleans. Sister Ramona reminded him that he should never disobey a nun. But he said, "No go."

Sister Ramona went out to the car. I tried to talk with Robert, but he remained adamantly opposed to any help.

When I stepped outside to make a phone call, I saw Sister Ramona talking to three kids around the car. She was giving away my dirty clothes! She had mistaken them for a bag of giveaway clothes.

I hastily retrieved my clothes, then made a phone call to headquarters to inform them of Robert's refusal. They were making calls to link him with the hospice. I stepped back inside and told Robert what was going on and explained that we'd return in an hour or so.

We had just left to visit the next client when I received a call from headquarters saying the hospice was on the way to Robert's. We turned back to tell Robert. When we arrived at his house, we found a note stuck in the door saying he'd gone to Biloxi VA Hospital.

I called the hospital three hours later, but they had no record of him. Sister Ramona reminded me that he was where he wanted to be, wherever that might be. She reminded me that we were there to help and that we can only do our best with what we have.

Then she reminded me to keep my eye out for donations. Always doing good and helping people.

On another day, I rode in an emergency response vehicle through Gautier with Rich, from Long Island, and Eileen and Arlene, twins from Alaska. Rich was a character, a man in his mid-50s with a sardonic sense of humor—a good match for me. I rode shotgun. As we drove through Gautier, we listened to Arlene and Eileen. Their banter sounded like that of a married couple. While they handed out meals, I went door-to-door to assess needs and quickly got seven referrals, mostly medical.

Our first visit was with Debbie, who had metastatic breast cancer. Her husband had a spinal cord injury and was paralyzed. When we walked in, we found her home health aide crying. She had an abscessed tooth and was in terrible pain. She had been trying all morning to find a dentist. Could things get any worse? Yes, they could.

Debbie and her husband lived in a beautiful log cabin on the bayou. But now it had mold growing on the walls and concrete floor and had been condemned.

Debbie cried as she met us. She told us she was part of a FEMA investigation. It started, according to Debbie, when she called to find out about the delay in getting a FEMA trailer that would accommodate her disabled husband. She was told that it had been delivered and signed for. Her call triggered an investigation and now she was frightened that there'd be some "retribution." Also, she needed to get to a hospital for her chemo.

I made some calls to headquarters for the immediate needs of Debbie and her home health aide, and then made a call regarding her trailer. I would never find out the outcome of my efforts and soon learned that was the norm for volunteering here. We would do what we could and then head on to the next stop.

We had a pleasant visit with someone who called himself the Plastic Man, a retired military man living in a formerly beautiful home on the bayou. His wife had gone to live with their son in Houston, but the Plastic Man stayed. We asked how he got his name. He told us he made planters and other tchotchkes from plastic pipe. He was amazingly upbeat and optimistic. Rich bought a flamingo from him.

Then we visited Pink Flamingo Man, who lived in a FEMA trailer next to the rubble that had formerly been three separate houses: his home, his parents' home, and his grandparents' home. His trailer was festooned with pink flamingo lights and other flamingo lawn ornaments. Pink Flamingo Man insisted on having us in for coffee, even though we told him we had coffee in the emergency response vehicle. After the storm, he had scrounged through the debris and found some mismatched cups and saucers. He resolutely served his guests "on the good china."

We sat on tree stumps and trailer steps overlooking the beautiful, and now calm, Gulf of Mexico at sunset. We were in the middle of all the debris, and there was nothing left. Even the rebar, the steel bars intended to reinforce concrete structures, were bent and snapped. But this gentleman's Southern hospitality prevailed, and his spirit was unbroken. This was his home and he had no intention of leaving.

So much graciousness and optimism. It left me wondering, *How would I have reacted to losing absolutely everything?* But it also left me knowing that we are more resilient that we ever think we are. Working in the post–Hurricane Katrina recovery had been awesome, in the truest sense of the word.

The Day My World Started Turning Faster

~

Christine Tebaldi, RN, MSN, PMHNP-BC

THERE HAVE BEEN many significant events that alter the landscape of our history. My father speaks about the radio broadcast President Roosevelt made when referring to the bombing of Pearl Harbor as "a day that will live in infamy." I have heard people comment on what they were doing when they learned that President Kennedy had been shot. People my own age share our stories of where we were when we first heard about the events that occurred on September 11, 2001. Images and emotions of so many historical moments emblazoned into our memories.

The events of 9/11 have incredibly deep meaning for many. For me, it is not only the sharing in the emotion of our nation, it also marks the advent of my disaster response work.

My role as an inpatient psychiatric nurse practitioner in Rochester, New York, was fairly new at the time. I had been working at a hospital for several years in the Psych Department, but had just transitioned to this new role. I could never have imagined how much more transition lay ahead.

When the news reports flashed, my coworkers and I were stunned. I recall a tremendous feeling of angst and distress coupled with disbelief and awe as I stood side by side with patients and staff alike.

Later, many noted that the repeated news broadcasts, playing the same devastating scenes over and over, were traumatic in and of themselves. But on that day, we continued to watch together. Together was the key.

Hospitals and healthcare agencies across the nation, especially in the Northeast, were gearing up to respond in any way possible. Whenever I think about that time, the first person I associate with the experience is a dear friend and colleague who happened to be standing close by in the conference room when the news hit. Her calm, cool, and collected demeanor was a stabilizing factor. Maintaining grace under fire is something to strive for during a crisis. In the weeks, months, and years to come, I would find out what it really means to achieve that state—or not.

They say out of crisis opportunity is born. Like so many others, I wanted to do something, anything. Life felt so uncertain and out of control. After I connected with family and friends, watched countless hours of news programming, participated in community responses such as candlelight vigils, and donated blood, I wanted to do something more.

I was aware that some colleagues were involved with our local American Red Cross chapter as part of a disaster mental health team. I knew very little about its role and mission, but I moved forward nonetheless.

I put in my volunteer application not knowing what would come next. Deployments and mobilization trainings were occurring in record numbers, and a few weeks after the events I was called.

My employer was extraordinarily supportive, and before I knew it, I was scheduled to go. There was a long to-do list. Volunteer badge? Check. Red Cross materials and pretraining? Check. Check. Bag packed, coverage at work found, friends and family notified? Check. Check. Check!

Then, just as I was ready to go, a close friend suffered the loss of her spouse. I was faced with the dilemma of whether to stay and offer my support, and possibly lose any opportunity for deployment, or just continue with my plans. After a roller coaster of emotions, I decided that I needed to stay home and support my friend. As it turned out, my deployment timeline was able to be adjusted.

I boarded a plane to Philadelphia for what is called mobilization training: a two-day training period designed to give you as much of the necessary information and skills as possible to prepare you for a disaster assignment.

The group was very anxious. Our instructors were wonderful, likely applying their own disaster mental health skills on us.

None of us knew whether we would actually be deployed to New York. Anxiety was running high. Every volunteer wanted to get to Ground Zero and help in any way we could. There were several disaster operations simultaneously occurring around the nation. Most were related to the terrorists' acts on September 11, but some were part of a response to natural disasters elsewhere in the country. I was among those assigned to the disaster operation at the World Trade Center in New York City.

I'll never forget that train ride to New York City. The crowded car was filled not only with people but with anticipation. The sense of uncertainty was palpable. What was it going to be like? What type of assignments would we get? Would we do a good job?

The experience was extremely humbling. My small contribution in one of the respite centers near the World Trade Center was a learning experience. The greatest of the lessons was how to maintain a compassionate presence: the ability to simply sit with a person and listen rather than talk, to "be" rather than "do."

Our work was with law enforcement, firefighters, construction and utility workers, and other disaster response volunteers. Many of these individuals shared their experience: long hours, intense work, being away from family and friends, the smells in the air, the hard hats, changing assignments, and simply what it was like just to keep working. In fact, many couldn't bring themselves to stop working.

While their stories are not mine to tell, I can offer that I felt extremely honored and, at times, overwhelmed being part of the response and recovery process.

Our interventions were often very simple. We never knew which interaction might be the one that really made a difference. Offering tissues, a bottle of water, or some much needed information could create a large impact in an instant. We approached each encounter in a compassionate way and attempted to meet the needs of that person directly affected by the disaster, the first responder, or our fellow volunteers. As a colleague said to me, "Isn't that why we got into healthcare work, to help people?"

Disaster mental health is a subset of disaster responders, generally licensed mental health professionals with specific training on how to apply clinical skills in a disaster setting. The work recognizes that there are several phases of disaster: anticipation, the immediate impact of the event, the immediate aftermath, a surge of support and response, a subsequent letdown, and then a rebuilding phase.

Emergencies and disasters can often be managed by local resources. In the event that the scale of the event is too large, additional state and federal resources will be deployed.

There are aspects of disaster and emergency work that settle in your spirit. One thing that makes an emergency or disaster response worker effective is his or her ability to move quickly from task to task and interaction to interaction and, most importantly, to prioritize and reprioritize.

Effective personnel generally do not show much emotion during the disaster itself. It's important to well-being and prevention of burnout to take good care of yourself and to do an introspective review of your work as soon as you are able.

Upon my return, I became more involved in our local American Red Cross chapter, as well as at the hospital where I was employed. I had the opportunity to encounter many disaster activities, including responding to two bus accidents, working in shelters related to an ice storm with widespread power outages, pandemic flu preparation, mobilization trainings for Hurricanes Katrina and Wilma, education consultations, coordinating team involvement, local fire response, and service to the armed forces.

I became a trainer for the chapter and joined colleagues in teaching disaster preparedness for the state of Iowa. To say that my initial disaster response experience in New York has shaped my professional life is an understatement. My work even changed to a clinical and leadership role in an emergency psychiatric setting, and I recognized a natural synergy between my professional and volunteer activities.

Whenever there is a local or national disaster, I have a sense that I should be a part of it. There certainly have been times when my professional or personal responsibilities have precluded me from responding. While it is always the correct decision not to deploy if you cannot perform optimally, those are actually the hardest choices for me. Although I have volunteered during many local disasters, 9/11 is the only national disaster I have responded to. I also have co-instructed mobilization classes for other volunteers.

Each deployment for me has some key similarities: The anticipation of what response will be needed. Rapid coordination of the actual response needed, which often requires a choice between staying with family and friends versus responding to the hospital or community. Long hours, chaos, downtime, variable leadership structures, and changing priorities.

My disaster response work after 9/11 initiated a long series of interests and events in my personal and professional life, leading me to where I am now. My world started turning at record speed. I'm still working in an emergency psychiatric setting and volunteering with disaster mental health services. And I have become better at tending to my own spirit. In so doing, I hope to continue this valuable work.

Hunting the Lion That Swallowed You

~

Mark A. Montijo, PhD

I WOULD LIKE TO begin by saying that I approach this subject with a great humbleness and a deep respect. Bad things do indeed happen, and I have seen firsthand the devastation this world sometimes has to offer. I have seen people crushed by it, and I have also had the great privilege to witness the courage of people who have overcome unthinkable loss.

At 4:31 A.M. on January 17, 1994, a magnitude 6.7 earthquake rocked the epicenter of Reseda, California, and the greater Los Angeles area. Damage occurred up to 85 miles away, with the most severe damage in the west San Fernando Valley and the cities of Santa Monica, Simi

Valley, and Santa Clarita. Eleven hospitals suffered structural damage and were forced to transfer patients. It was estimated that 72 people died as a result of the quake, and more than 9,000 were injured. The quake caused an estimated $20 billion in damage, then one of the costliest natural disasters in U.S. history.

At the time, I was working as an Employee Assistance Program (EAP) coordinator providing crisis intervention, as well as family and addictions counseling for my company's employees. I lived about four miles from the epicenter. That morning, I was awakened by a violent shaking that knocked my home off its foundation. Frightened and confused, I didn't know what had happened until I made my way through the fallen debris in my home, got outside, and turned on my car radio. It was very cold and dark. Up and down the street, my neighbors were standing outside their homes in pajamas and nightgowns, shaken and confused. I shut off the natural-gas line into my home, as well as the electricity.

Later that morning, I drove to my company's administration building located closer to my home instead of my own office. I knew that all the company's leaders would be gathered there and I needed to check in with them. The electricity was out all over the San Fernando Valley, so none of the traffic lights worked. I carefully eased my way through the intersections. My gas gauge read about a quarter of a tank. This concerned me, as the gas pumps were out as well. None of the phones worked, and my mobile phone worked only sporadically. Over the radio, it was announced that the water system may have been compromised; tap water was not safe to drink. Later I discovered that my own office building had been "red tagged" as unsafe, and I was unable to recover any records or supportive material.

I walked into the local office and attended a hastily arranged meeting at which I learned of the extensive damage to the company's buildings and the resultant impact on the services our company provides to the public. I also began a search to secure and supply an office from which I could organize counseling for the thousands of employees who were affected. I commandeered an empty conference room inside a larger building, borrowed a desk, a chair, and a phone, and set up camp. As I sat for a moment in the borrowed chair surveying my makeshift office, I felt the earthquake's frightening aftershock.

I needed help. Eventually, I was able to get through to my national office in Washington, D.C., and set the stage for additional counselors to fly in from out of the immediate area.

And so began the months' long process of counseling those who had been affected by the quake. This I did in groups and one-on-one meetings. In this kind of situation, you don't always get to meet with people in an appropriate setting. Often, a storage room or janitor's closet has to substitute for a consult room. On many occasions, debriefing occurred right on the workroom floor, and I would have to create a feeling of privacy while people were working all around us. Sometimes there were

aftershocks in the middle of these sessions, causing everyone to jump up and anxiously glance around at the walls
and ceiling. I got used to checking for quick escape routes
as I chose my seat. I also got into the habit of scanning
every building I entered for cracks in the walls or floor,
possible evidence of structural damage.

As I settled into the rhythm of conducting one counseling session after another, I soon learned that those at
greatest risk were the ones who had already been trying
as hard as they could to stay afloat psychologically prior
to the quake. Also severely affected were those who had
experienced previous trauma, especially during war; the
quake and its aftershocks were eerily similar to bombs or
artillery exploding. One man I spoke with told me the
damaged buildings reminded him of the bombed-out
buildings "at home." Then he broke down and began to
cry. I also met with a middle-aged, normally high-func-
tioning man who couldn't sleep inside his home with his
family. He slept in the driver's seat of his car, parked in
his driveway, with a loaded gun on his lap. One young
woman who had climbed her way out of a collapsed apartment building was haunted by images of a dusty darkness
sharply punctuated by flashlight beams and the cries of
those who were trapped.

We had all imagined that the life we lived would continue unchanged; we took many things for granted. The
assumptions of everyone who had been affected by the
quake had been shattered. When I went to sleep the night
of the quake, I assumed that I would awaken without

incident, just as I assumed that I would have dinner that evening at home around 6:00 P.M., as usual. I no longer make those types of assumptions. Natural disasters are a jarring reminder that we are not in control. Unexpected events shatter our assumptive world of reason, order, and constancy, and force upon us the restructuring of a new worldview that includes those new and different possibilities. This can be a long and psychologically arduous process. I now know why my father would preface any statement about the future with, "God willing and the creek don't rise."

There has been much argument about the best way to proceed in the aftermath of a traumatic event. I feel strongly that in the immediate aftermath, simple wisdom should prevail. Disaster researchers Richard Gist and S. Joseph Woodall concluded in their study of the origins and natural history of debriefing that the most important lessons to guide helping efforts in times of turmoil came more from Grandma than from grad school: "People are resilient; friends are important; conversation helps; time is a great healer; look out for others while you look out for yourself."

Keeping in mind that human beings are naturally resilient, a pragmatic approach is called for; basic needs such as safety, food, and shelter are paramount and should be considered first and foremost. The ability to communicate with loved ones via cell phone or other means can be calming and healing. Accurate information about what occurred (who, what, where, and why) during the traumatic event should be made available as soon as possible so that people can begin the long process of incorporating the facts into their knowledge base and integrating them emotionally. We must acknowledge that people heal in their own way. Lastly, the community at large should acknowledge that something of great significance has happened.

Looking back, I see that I too was traumatized by my experience during the quake. After a long day of debriefing clients, I would return home, fall asleep in my clothes (after all, you never know if you might have to run out of the house), and get up to do it all over again the next day. Trying to identify what was happening to me would have been like trying to hunt the lion that had already swallowed me: I was too immersed in it to see it. As caregivers, it is important to acknowledge that the destruction wrought by traumatic events spreads beyond those who were there to include those who experienced it vicariously. As mental health practitioners, we collect bits and pieces of accounts of trauma. The cumulative effect of chronic exposure to the traumatic images of our patients can have an impact on our worldview, our personal relationships, and our sense of self. This can lead to cynicism and even despair.

It is important that mental health professionals maintain self-awareness and monitor for signs of burnout. Proactive measures are best. When signs of burnout or stress are noticeable, it's already too late. Commonsense suggestions include: stay connected with colleagues, seek consultation if needed, maintain balance between work and play, maintain physical and spiritual activities, and add humor to your life every day.

Professionals who deal with trauma need to remember that although bad things do indeed happen, there is a lot of good in the world too. We also see that we are interconnected with one another much more than we had ever dreamed. In times of despair, people rally with great courage and sacrifice, and our families and loved ones are most important.

Be Prepared

~

Richard Rhodes

IT WAS AUGUST, Friday the 13th. The state of Florida was preparing for Hurricane Charley, a storm that by all accounts was heading for the Tampa Bay area. I took up position in what I thought would be a good location to serve in my role as a Regional Emergency Response Advisor (RERA) for the Florida Department of Health. That morning I left my home in Punta Gorda and went to the Charlotte County Emergency Operations Center, where I could monitor the storm and coordinate with my local emergency management agency on storm preparation for the northern counties in my region. I was responsible for advising ten county health departments in southwestern Florida on health and medical emergency support

operations and acted as a liaison between the state and
county Emergency Operations Centers (EOC).

I arrived at the Charlotte County center around eight
o'clock that morning. It seemed like a normal August day,
warm and humid, with some high clouds streaming across
the sky. Nothing about the conditions outside suggested
there was anything stirring out in the Gulf of Mexico.

When I entered the building and signed the sign-in
sheet, I noticed very little activity. Other local agencies
were starting to arrive for the morning situation briefing.
As I entered into the crowded main room of the EOC, I
looked up at the satellite pictures of Charley being pro-
jected onto the wall. Charley was looking good coming
off the tip of Cuba, but it wasn't all that powerful a storm.
It was still a Category 1, and the National Hurricane
Center still had it approaching the Tampa Bay area in the
evening to early morning hours.

As the briefing started, Wayne Sallade, Charlotte
County emergency manager, talked about the current situation, then went around the room asking each agency to
provide an update of its current preparatory actions. I was
sitting at a table designated for state responders and had
my own laptop with the satellite and radar views rolling
over and over, hypnotized by the continual loop of clouds
and colors.

My family—my wife, four kids, and two dogs—was
at our home in Punta Gorda. After the briefing, I got
a Nextel direct connect from my oldest son, Andrew, a

curious soon-to-be 11-year-old. "Beep beep," the direct connect sounded.

"Dad, are you there?"

I pushed the button. "Yeah, what's up?"

"I just wanted to see what you're doing."

"Nothing," I said. He proceeded to let me know that he was worried because the dogs were acting weird. Not knowing what would happen next, I told him everything was fine.

At about 10:30 A.M., I started to notice a slight track change to the radar loop of Charley. It's normal for a storm to wobble left or right of the track, but I thought I might start watching it a little more closely. Charley had also gained strength by this time and was quickly approaching Category 2 strength. A few minutes later, my son beeped me again.

"Dad, it looks like the storm is moving toward us."

I explained that it sometimes appears that way but not to worry, that if he was worried it was going to hit us, he should do some things to help get his mind off it. I had him put a mattress in the hallway of our home, as this is the only area with no windows or exterior walls. I told him that if it comes, that will be a safe place to hang out. It would be kind of like playing fort.

By 11:00 A.M. the writing was on the wall. Hurricane Charley was changing course, despite the Hurricane Center continuing to forecast a direct hit on Tampa. The 11:00 A.M. advisory had Hurricane Charley as a full Category 2 storm and strengthening. By now the direct-connect communication with my son was nonstop every ten minutes. He was very frightened and wanted to evacuate.

I started to feel some concern myself, as I had taken no precautionary measures to protect my family or home. My wife had, though. She'd stocked up on water and canned goods and was in the process of clearing the yard of anything that could be blown around. It was my responsibilities that had been neglected.

You see, my job always came first; my family was second. I am often haunted by this fact. I was more willing to prepare the citizens for the storm than I was to help prepare my own family. My wife did the brunt of that work. For the life of me, I cannot figure out why she has stuck by me for so long.

At 12:15 P.M. and after numerous calls from Andrew, I talked to my wife, Carol. We both agreed that they were not going to a local shelter because it did not take pets. The dogs were a part of the family, and we would not leave them any more than we would leave our kids.

At the next emergency management briefing, Wayne made it clear that he was planning for a direct hit. "We have to evacuate the EOC and keep minimal manning here. We will be running the operation out of the Charlotte County Jail," he announced. Then he told us that while the storm was a Cat-2, a Category 2, and the current Emergency Operations Center was rated for a Cat-3, he needed to plan for a Cat-4. That is an emergency management rule: always plan one category higher than predicted. He told us that he did not have room for everyone, and that we needed to keep the staffing to a minimum. I consulted the local health department, and they were going to continue to man the Emergency Support Functions desk for the county.

After the briefing, at around 12:30 P.M., I contacted the State Health Department Emergency Support Functions desk in the State Emergency Operations Center. I reached my good friend Sam MacDonnell.

"Sam, it's me, Rick. Hey, the local center here in Charlotte is going to COOP [Continuity of Operation Plan] to the jail, and there is not enough space there for me."

"Okay," Sam replied.

"I am heading out and will be running operations from my home. I can set up the satellite phone and communication in case we lose power and phone lines. I'll keep you posted," I said, then hung up. Five minutes later, as I walked out to my truck and pulled a drag off my cigarette, my phone rang. It was Sam.

"What's up, brother? Wasn't the last call enough?"

I heard concern in his voice as he answered, "Rick, the locals don't know this yet, but Charley has jumped from a Cat-2 to a Cat-4 storm and is heading straight for you and Punta Gorda. It looks like it's coming right up the harbor."

I remember my exact response: "Shit!"

"Ray wants you to take the state response vehicle and get out of there, now!" Sam replied.

I told Sam I was not leaving without my family. I could hear him having a side conversation with someone and assumed it was Ray Runo, our boss. He came back on and told me that Ray authorized me to load the family in the response vehicle and get out of town. By now it was close to 1:30 P.M.

I called Carol and broke in before she could speak. "Get whatever is near and dear to you and throw it in a trash bag. I am going to pull in the driveway and you are going to get in and we are getting out of here," I said. She could tell I was scared and all she said was, "Okay."

"I am five minutes away, so you have that much time," I barked.

By now the rain had started to fall. My concern was to find a hotel and not get stuck in traffic. As I pulled into the driveway, my wife and kids, the two oldest with a dog in their arms, ran out to the Chevy Tahoe with its lights and sirens going. I jumped out and popped the rear hatch. I had a ton of response equipment in the back, but we managed to get a large trash bag full of pictures and important documents into the truck, along with a couple of dog crates. The four kids piled in a backseat made for three, and my wife sat up front with me.

Off we went!

As we crossed the state of Florida, on back roads to avoid heavy traffic, the winds and rain began to sweep in. I had the response radio in my truck tuned in to the news and weather station so we could listen for warnings and take shelter if need be. Not that there are an abundance of places to shelter on State Road 70 from Arcadia to Fort Pierce.

By now Carol's and my nerves were frazzled. We cracked the windows of the vehicle, and I lit a cigarette. My phone rang.

"Rick," Sam said. "The roof on the shelter in Arcadia has blown off. It is unknown if there are any injuries."

I had the phone on speaker so that I could drive and talk at the same time. I said to Carol, "Damn, I think there were about 15 hundred people in that shelter. This is not good!"

We started making phone calls looking for hotels in Fort Pierce. All were full. I called my dad in Jacksonville. "I know this is going to be weird, but can you call Uncle Phil in Vero Beach and see if we can stay with him?"

It was weird because aside from the occasional email when I was in Iraq, my "Uncle" Phil and I had not talked to or seen each other in 20 years. Now I was asking him if I could drop my family and dogs at his house for an indefinite period of time. And he isn't even a blood uncle, but rather a close friend of my dad.

My father called me back and said that Phil had no problem with housing us. As we drove from Fort Pierce to Vero Beach, we could hear the reports coming across AM talk radio. It didn't sound good for the folks left in Punta Gorda.

When we arrived at my uncle's house, he came out to greet us with open arms. He really was a great and hospitable man. We unloaded and then went into town

to get something to eat. When we got back, we were trying to catch up on the damage to our town by watching
local news. Uncle Phil did not have cable, so the pictures
we saw through the static of his rabbit ear reception were
hard to make out. But it was clear that Punta Gorda and
Port Charlotte had taken a hit.

We all lay down early in the evening, physically and
mentally drained. It was then that I had time to think.
Could all of this have been avoided? Of course the storm
could not have been, but my preparedness and taking care
of my family could have been. Was I going to be able to
focus on the response and serving people when I was worried about my wife and kids, our home, our belongings?
The answer was no.

About midnight I got a call from Mike Jacobs in the
South East Operations Center. Mike said that the devastation was exceptional and that they needed me on the
road now to get back to Punta Gorda. I kissed my wife
and off I went on what should have been about a two-
hour trek back across the state. It took several hours. I did
not get back to Punta Gorda until about 5:00 A.M.

The storm had left Arcadia in rubble. As I drove
down US 17 from Arcadia to Punta Gorda, the debris told
the story. I did not expect to have a home left, and my
mind focused strictly on that fact. What were we going
to do? I could not go to work until I saw the damage that
had been done to my home and could let Carol know.

By driving through ditches, over downed power lines,
and through fields, I made it to my neighborhood. I had

to take the last half-mile by foot because I could not get in with the vehicle.

I grabbed my flashlight out of the truck and proceeded down the dark and eerily quiet street. A dog passed in front of me, and it looked as if it had spent the whole storm outside. As I made it to my driveway, the house looked different from all the others. There was no visible damage! I walked around to the back and, again, there was nothing. Shining my light on the roof, the windows, the doors, and all around, I found nothing wrong or out of place. My neighbor's roof had some damage; the houses down the road were missing roofs—but mine, nothing. I fell to my knees, tears rolling down my face, and asked what I had done to deserve this fortune.

The next two weeks would be full of stories of their own, but this one provided me with a lesson that I often use when instructing responders. It is our duty to make sure that we are prepared to assist the public we serve. If we are not prepared, our families are not prepared. How can we expect others, who don't know better, to be prepared?

If I'd had a family preparedness plan and my family had been my priority, it would have taken a load off my mind. I could then have focused on my job. I would not have been worried about my home because I'd have done what I could to protect it. I would not have been worried about my family, because they would have known where and when to leave. Having a family plan and making your family the number-one priority are like insurance. They will give you the peace of mind that you need in order to serve the public.

In the Dust of 9/11

~

Sally Roy-Boynton, *DBA, MSN, ARNP*

WHEN I VOLUNTEERED to go to New York City after 9/11 as a Red Cross disaster mental health worker, my family and friends could not understand why. "Don't you know you might be putting yourself in harm's way?" they asked. At the time no one was sure when the next terrorist attack might occur.

As I prepared for the trip from my home in Dubuque, Iowa, my family expressed concerns about my safety and maybe even my sanity for wanting to volunteer for this humanitarian effort.

"I want to be part of history," I responded. "I want to help. I don't know what I'll do, or with who, but whatever happens to me, I will know that I did my part."

I've never regretted my decision to go, and the years since have not blurred the memories. This was the most dramatic look at suffering and inhumanity that I've ever experienced.

No, I did not work at Ground Zero. I was assigned to a service center many blocks away, on the edge of Chinatown. Daily, hundreds of individuals who had lost their jobs or homes or suffered in some way from the tragedy came seeking assistance. Some needed food, some housing, some medical care or medications, or other items too numerous to mention.

Chinatown was on the outskirts of Ground Zero and had lost power for many days. Many of the businesses in that part of the city were restaurants, and they had lost all their food. In addition, they were dependent on tourism, which had come to a grinding halt. The people of Chinatown suffered personal and financial losses.

Logistically, the service center was too small to hold the hundreds of people who came on a daily basis to seek help. And, in reality, there were only enough case workers to complete applications on approximately 100 individuals a day. Applicants waiting for help lined the sidewalks outside the building from daybreak to well past dark. Many would not get to meet with a worker, would not get help that day, and would have to come back and try again the next day.

Each morning at 7:00 A.M., as I stepped out of the subway stairs, I saw hundreds waiting on the sidewalk in front of and beside the service center. The workers' first job of the day would be to go out, make lines, and count off 150 individuals. The rest would be told there was no use waiting. "Come back another day, or go to another service center," they were told. This news understandably brought anger, frustration, and distress to those who had to leave.

A striking reality of my assignment was that, two weeks after the event, the air was still heavy with smoke, stench, and soot. People wore masks if working at, or even walking near, Ground Zero. But even many blocks away at the service center, the air quality was not much better. The air was irritating to the nose, throat, lungs, and eyes. Every day my eyes burned, and I constantly blew blood from my irritated nose.

The large dump trucks used to haul debris away from Ground Zero had to be washed to prevent the toxic dust from being taken into the city. I thought it odd to see small children playing on the swings and teeter-totters at the school just across the street from the wash station.

The air quality sensors mounted on the telephone poles and levels were read daily by city workers. The levels reported in the newspaper assured us over and over that there was nothing toxic or dangerous in the air. Months later, after my return home, however, I received a request from the federal government and the Red Cross. They wanted to study the long-term effects of the air quality on the volunteers!

"How bizarre," I thought. *I was there only two months. I wonder if they are testing the people who live there.*

My job as a disaster mental health worker was to talk to the persons waiting to be seen and to assess whether they had mental health issues or were experiencing any posttraumatic stress syndrome symptoms. This may sound relatively simple for a nurse who has been in the mental health field for 20-plus years. But 95 percent of those waiting did not speak English! The service center had a battery of volunteer interpreters, but there were so many languages and so many dialects that it was rare to be able to match up a client with an interpreter.

I reverted to the basics of mental health nursing: meeting people's physical needs for food, fluids, and warmth. I passed out blankets and, on rainy days, ponchos. I tried to make people comfortable. Some sat on the sidewalk, some on chairs from the service center.

A friendly smile or gentle touch was all that some folks needed; others were frustrated and angry, and nothing could fill their emptiness. For the children there were stuffed animals to be given out. Schoolchildren from all over the United States had sent cards, letters, and items they thought people might need.

Those individuals who could speak English would spend the hours waiting and retelling their personal stories about September 11. Some had pictures to show, others just had the pictures in their minds and the memories of the screams as people they knew jumped from the windows of the towers.

Survival guilt was all too common. Stories of "why I wasn't at work that day" and how "the person who replaced me is now dead" weighed heavily on people's minds.

I talked one day with a woman who was returning daily to her apartment near Ground Zero to water her flowers and plants with bottled water that she carried through the checkpoints. "I know if my plants can survive down there, someday I can go back and survive there, too," she told me.

One fellow told me he came to New York after the flood disaster in Houston to find work; now his work was again taken away by this disaster. "What will you do next?" I asked. He wasn't sure, but he was quite sure he was not going to stay in New York City.

Age, wealth, and affluence had no preference in the waiting line at the service center. There were people young and old. There were those in rags and those in minks. Disaster had affected each individual's life in some manner.

At the end of each day, physically exhausted and emotionally drained, I took the subway back to my hotel near Times Square. The walk from the subway to the hotel was several blocks. It was a time to unwind and process my thoughts on the day. I took time each night to write in a journal some of my thoughts about what I was seeing and experiencing. Family pictures I had brought along reminded me how lucky I was and made me thankful I could return to my comfortable home.

I had Thanksgiving dinner that year in New York, compliments of donations from the Red Cross workers. It was wonderful, but my heart was heavy for what I was seeing and experiencing. In years since, Thanksgiving has had a totally different meaning for me than it ever had.

Life in general has a different meaning. I no longer take my health, my circumstances, or my life for granted. I am witness to how quickly people's lives can be turned upside down and circumstances changed forever.

I'm glad I volunteer. I've worked for victims of natural disasters, plane crashes, and many types of tragedies, but the 9/11 disaster is the one that most shaped my perspective on life and the fragile circumstances that we exist in each day.

Holistic Care in the Eye of the Storm

~

Scharmaine Lawson-Baker,
DNP, FNP–BC

T HE STORY OF my life can be categorized into three phases: pre-Katrina, Katrina, and post-Katrina. I believe these classifications fit the lives of many New Orleanians, who undeniably went through the worst natural disaster ever to hit the United States.

I am a native of New Orleans, known for its toe-tapping music, jaw-dropping architecture, and mouth-watering restaurants and also for Mardi Gras and those haunted above ground cemeteries. I lived in the city until 1991 and, after living as a travel nurse in several states and countries, I returned in 2001 to, as my grandma would say, "put some roots down."

As a board-certified family nurse practitioner, placing my "roots" led me to launch Advanced Clinical Consultants in the spring of 2005. During this phase of my life, my newly formed house-call practice was blossoming as fast as the daffodils were peeking through the dirt. We had risen from 15 to 100 patients in just four months and had several physicians supporting the practice. I prided myself on having a 24- to 48-hour turnaround for admission to my house-call practice, once I received a referral. Our practice is geared toward the elderly, bedbound, and disabled patients who would otherwise not receive primary care services. I was enjoying the early fruits of success, including total autonomy and a growing clientele.

Then on August 27, 2005, we were asked to evacuate New Orleans—yet again. We had left just a couple of months earlier for Hurricane Ivan, only to return home a few days afterward because it turned out to be only a scare.

On the morning of the Katrina evacuation, the air was still and the clouds were slightly overcast as I anxiously packed the same two shirts, slippers, and toothbrush I had packed a couple of months before and hit the road. I casually grabbed my personal digital assistant (PDA), thinking that this might actually be the Big One. That device would literally save my practice.

Hurricane Katrina changed my life and the lives of all of my patients forever. It would be three long months before I would be able to return home from my hiatus in

San Antonio. While in the Lone Star state, I was miraculously able to keep the lines of communication open with families of my patients and reach several people who were scattered across all 50 states, thanks to my PDA! I was able to speak with nurses, physicians, and other healthcare personnel who phoned me regarding some of my patients they were caring for.

For instance, I had a physician contact me from Idaho who was taking care of one of my patients at a local shelter. The physician was not able to ascertain the appropriate medication list or find out if the patient was up-to-date on her mammogram. I was able to pull this information from my PDA and give it to him over the phone.

There was another case in which the family of one of my patients called looking for their mother and brother, who had refused to evacuate their ninth Ward home. The caller said he was speaking to his mother as the water rose to her waist, and he wanted to know if I had heard anything. Well, as a matter of fact, I had; I had just spoken with a hospice director in Kansas who was inquiring about his mother's laboratory results. I was able to connect several families by acting as a liaison between the missing and the searching during this time.

This was very rewarding because I was able to provide assistance even though I was not caring for the patients in the form of house calls. I was able to provide emotional and social support, dimensions that are easily overlooked. I was also able to find comfort in dealing with my own tremendous loss, uncertainty, and frustration by helping others to connect. After weeks of helping many families reunite, I began to heal and feel a sense of worth. Therefore, every time I was able to help a distant physician, frightened family member, or scared patient, my burdens felt a little lighter.

Three months after Hurricane Katrina, I returned to New Orleans and discovered that our neighborhood was still accessible only by boat. The office building was gone and all charts were clumped together by a thick slosh of greenish mud. I had no other choice but to totally rebuild and start the practice all over again. While rebuilding the gutted office, I worked out of a 500-square-foot, one-bedroom apartment for weeks until I was finally able to move in on June 1, 2006. My PDA came to the rescue once again, as I was able to retrieve information on all my patients from its database. Sadly, most of them had been killed in the flood or displaced to another state.

I was one of only a handful of local providers who had returned to find their patients and rebuild their practices. My phone rang off the hook for weeks. The lack of primary care providers and the constant stream of people returning to the city led to a surge in patients for my practice. The boost in patients was also the result of the downed hospital systems and the lack of transportation for many people returning home.

My practice swelled to 500 patients within six months of my return home. I purchased an electronic medical record (EMR) because my PDA was no longer able to accommodate the volume. I am convinced that it was because of my usage of health information technology (HIT) that I was able to hit the ground running after the disaster, whereas other physicians and major hospitals experienced a delay because of lost documents. Later, I would be called upon to provide more than medical care.

Holistic care was something I had always practiced. I prided myself on treating the whole person, but I'm not so sure I actually realized how all the dimensions affect one another. For example, one patient had poorly controlled hypertension and was on five blood pressure drugs, but still presented with consistently elevated blood pressure readings. After a long talk with him, I discovered that he was upset because he had yet to get through to FEMA to get a trailer. He explained that he had been calling every day and would only get a busy signal. He also said that he was tired and scared to stay in his gutted house. After making a few phone calls to get his FEMA trailer delivered to him, we noticed that we were able to wean him quickly from five to two blood pressure medications. Two weeks after receiving the precious FEMA trailer, he was off all antihypertensive medications. This underscores the importance of treating all dimensions of a person, because sometimes the cure is not in a pill.

Another case involved a 92-year-old woman who had Type II uncontrolled diabetes with really high blood sugar. I was titrating the insulin for weeks and had maxed out on all oral hypoglycemics (pills used to treat diabetes)—until she confided to me that her light bill was $2,500!

"HaMercy," is all I could say as I just stared at her.

"I don't know what I'm going to do," she said. Then she burst into tears.

After that statement, I noticed the thick orange power cord flowing across her front porch through her neighbor's torn screen door, and I knew I had to find a solution. I called our social worker and we managed to get her lights turned back on. The real reason she hadn't paid the bill was because her eyesight was so poor that she couldn't read it. It took several weeks, but after getting familial support and additional home resources, we weaned her off the insulin. Yet again, once the social needs are met, the physical body is healed.

We at Advanced Clinical Consultants only admit elderly, bedbound, and disabled patients to the practice, but I will go anywhere to see a client. This phenomenon has also contributed to the spike in clientele. I have been known to care for patients on their back porches, rooftops, attics, and in homes that have been stripped down and gutted to the studs. Have bag, will travel.

There has been a tremendous shortage of nurses, physicians, and every other healthcare professional in New Orleans since Hurricane Katrina. Most hospital emergency room waits are now three to four hours. With the mass return of people to New Orleans, I am not able to see patients fast enough. Instead of one-day or two-day turnarounds, I now have a two-week waiting list for non-emergency cases and a one-week waiting list for patients who need to be seen sooner. On average, I make approximately ten home visits a day, a sharp increase from my pre-Katrina schedule of five or six patients a day.

In addition to my EMR and tablet PC with detachable keyboard, I e-prescribe all my medications to the patients' pharmacy of choice. So I can prescribe to pharmacies across the city and even in other states, which is helpful during evacuation times.

The most important lesson I have learned from this devastating storm that ripped apart my life and the lives of my patients is to treat the "whole" person all the time. It has taught me to delve a little deeper during my history taking and to take a closer look at the subtleties that are often overlooked in a person's home. I am deeply committed to the rebirth of my fair Crescent City and honored to be back serving those who would otherwise not receive healthcare in their homes, while perfecting the art of holistic care.

Tsunami!

~

Marko Cunningham

As we approached Phuket, we came in low. The plane circled several times, so we were able to see miles of debris and what appeared to be bodies. It was the first real impression of the tsunami we had gotten, and everyone looked down upon the carnage in silence.

I am a volunteer fire/EMT officer for a Thai nongovernment organization in Bangkok. I had been called to go to Phuket to assist the injured and take care of the dead. It is part of the job.

We landed and exited the aircraft, but as we turned to find out where we should go next, we saw a large group of what appeared to be tourists walking across the airport fields. As they came closer, we noticed that they seemed to be injured and hobbling and that one person was being carried. As we walked toward them, we could see that they were indeed all injured and in need of assistance. We broke into a run. When we got close enough to see their faces, some looked shocked, some looked sad, some looked to be in pain. We made a makeshift shoe for one man, carried two others, and helped everyone else in whatever way we could.

I was the only one of our team who spoke English, so I was bombarded with questions, many of which I could not answer. My mind reeled as they described what had happened to them, their families, and their friends. I hopped on the back of a truck full of coffins, which I took at the time as an ominous sign, and we headed into Phuket. We arrived at Patong Hospital and set up in an unfinished hotel across the road. It had nothing inside but was spotlessly clean and new. We unpacked and then headed down to Patong beach for our first look at the damage.

The first body I saw was in a hotel, still full of water. We waded in and found a small boy floating on top of the water in one of the rooms, eyes bulging and lips swollen. It felt unreal. Maybe that was a blessing, because it helped me to handle the many bodies I would soon see. These things we were collecting no longer seemed human.

The day passed quickly and, though I got used to the sight of deformed bodies, my first trip to the makeshift morgue beneath the Patong Hospital was a gagging experience. The bodies reeked and it was hard to stomach, but I had no choice but to do the job as we placed the newly found corpses in the ever growing rows.

We returned to our rooms late in the evening. The next morning we were up early and out again. I was told to stick around the Patong area to help foreigners in the search for their missing relations and to help in identifying corpses, and I was a contact for foreign media on the scene.

One case in particular really affected me. A man came to the Ocean Plaza, which was being pumped of water. He asked me to help find his wife, who had been shopping in the plaza. I explained it would be a while before we could get inside. I didn't explain that there would be little chance of finding anyone alive.

Later, we did find a body that I was able to identify as this man's wife. I showed him the passport. He nodded and his shoulders dropped. The he looked up at me and said, "Thank you," and hugged me.

It was all I could do to stop the tears as they welled up in my eyes. I didn't know what to say or do and didn't quite understand why he was thanking me, so I just stood there, and then he gave me a little forced smile and walked away.

Suddenly, I dealt with the last two days in two seconds. All the bodies I had collected had names and faces and lives and families and sadness and pain. It was the worst part of the whole experience. I started to humanize the bodies, and I didn't like it. I had to avoid thinking about it, otherwise I couldn't survive to do the job.

On the evening of the second day, we left Patong and headed up the coast to Khao Lak. We arrived at a place called Watt Bang Muang at about 8:00 P.M. It is a name I will never forget.

I exited the van in the temple grounds, surrounded by tall trees visible only through a dim, yellow light emanating from a festoon of bulbs strung between trees. I was handed a pair of surgical gloves and a mask and told to help unload a large truck that had just arrived.

The first thing that struck me was the smell. My tired mind recoiled at the overpowering smell of death. I turned and followed my team as we walked toward the truck.

As I came closer, I stopped and stared in disbelief. I couldn't believe that there were so many bodies piled one on top of the other, like images of the Holocaust from a movie. If someone hadn't slapped me on the back and said, "Let's go, Marko," I believe I would still be there staring now.

I was unsure where to go, so I followed the guy who was helping me carry the first corpse. We walked toward a dark area in a field. As we approached, I looked in horror as I realized that this field was absolutely full of bodies. We put the body down in a row with many others, and I stood back and looked up and down the rows as far as I could see until the darkness swallowed them up. This must be what hell is like.

I can't remember how many bodies I helped carry that night. I can't remember the faces of the dead or what I talked about with people. I only remember that when I got back to the school where we were to sleep that night, I couldn't eat.

I retired to bed and lay awake thinking. Looking back, I realize I was in shock. I have seen and handled dead bodies often in my work, but the sheer volume made this different. I had to think of a reason to get out of this place! I thought of lying and saying that my father was sick and I needed to return home. I thought of many excuses during the night. I was desperate to get out of that hellhole. I was stunned. How could there be so many people dead?

I finally fell asleep on a concrete floor with sheets used to carry the dead as bedding. I woke up in the morning tired, but feeling different. I don't know what happened overnight. I just said to myself, "Okay, Marko. Let's get back to work." I realized that if I didn't do this work someone else would have to take my place, and I couldn't live with myself for doing that to someone else. I had joined this Thai group three years before and they had only recently started to accept me into their brotherhood. If I left now it would all be gone. I felt leaving would be even more difficult than staying here now.

We walked and began to kit up with gloves and basic cotton masks. A pickup pulled up and asked me to join them to go out for bodies. We went down to Khao Lak, which we had passed in the dark the night before. Now, in the daylight, things seemed even worse. I looked out across kilometers of fields that had once had villages and

luxurious hotels on them, but now nothing. Nothing! Just
the concrete slabs of flooring that outlined where a building once stood.

We jumped out of the truck and began to walk across the
fields, scanning the horizon for evidence of remains. It was
barren, but we knew there had once been a village here.

I looked far and wide until my eyes ached under the
strain of the midday sun. Then, in my peripheral vision, I
saw something sticking out of the mud. A glove? A hand?
It was the latter.

A human hand reached out of the ground toward me
as if asking for help. I shouted to the guys, and they ran
to me. As we inspected more carefully, we saw more and
more. We realized that the area was literally full of bodies! We were standing on a graveyard of people. One of
the volunteers called our boss to tell him. We thought we
had discovered an unusual thing, but soon learned this
was only one of many sites littered with the dead.

Our small group started to remove the bodies, one by
one, untangling them from the silt and debris that they
were entwined in. Soon our pickup was full. We wearily
climbed into the back of the truck in between the corpses
and rode away.

We arrived back at the temple and unloaded. My boss
found me and asked me to stay at the temple because foreigners were arriving and needed assistance. I knew no
one in our group spoke English and most were too shy to
approach foreigners, so it seemed a reasonable idea. I acted
as though I was disappointed, but in fact I didn't want to

go out into the fields again. It was a dirty, difficult job that I was glad to be relieved of. And in the days that followed, when things at the temple got worse and the smell became nearly unbearable and the maggots crawled over my feet and hands, I always thought to myself, *Better here than in the fields again!*

The only English speaker, I had a lot of unwanted responsibility in dealing with grieving relatives. That was the hardest part: dealing with the relatives. They were all so brave. They often asked me if I was okay. I thought it striking that in the midst of their loss, they were concerned for me.

I remember one man, a doctor who had come to the temple searching for his wife. I went through uncovering maybe 30 or 40 bodies from their sheet coffins, without success. He thanked me and asked if he could help in any way. He said he felt guilty for spending so much time looking for his wife when maybe he should be trying to help. He walked over to a pile of body sheets and sat on them, holding his head in his hands. I felt so sad for him. His story was just one of so many.

And slowly I began to be desensitized. After a few days, I had lost my sense of sadness and respect for the bodies that came in endlessly. The pickups came in all day long. I hated them. I was tired, as was everyone. Nerves were on edge. I woke up every morning, went to work, came home, ate, and collapsed on my body-bag bed.

Every morning there was an old lady on a motorcycle with a sidecar and a big pot of Kow Tom, rice porridge with pork. She fed us. No one knew who she was, or her story, but she was there every morning.

Outside in the field behind our school were two huge plastic water containers for showering. There were no walls, so we showered with briefs or boxers on, or waited until after dark. Everyone stopped shaving and our general appearance was getting low. In the beginning, I used Vicks under my nose in an attempt to ward off the smell of the bodies, but I was told by a more experienced body collector to just let it go, I would get used to it. He was right.

After a few days, the temple had swelled with bodies and volunteers. We now had some excellent translators, mostly students from Bangkok. Doctors and assistants were beginning DNA identification of the bodies. By the end of the first week, help arrived in the form of doctors and groups from many countries.

It had been a horrible job and no one, including myself, wanted to do it. At least that's what I thought at the time. I was to be proved wrong the day it came for me to leave.

Days rolled on. I heard from many friends in New Zealand via calls on my cell phone. When an interview was shown on TV news, my parents received calls from friends, family, and people they didn't even know, with words of praise for their son. It made them proud, and in turn that made what I was doing easier to handle. Just the feeling that someone was thinking of me and I was not alone made it better!

My father told me later that there was one elderly couple who called to say, "You must be so proud of your son." My father replied, "I have always been proud of him." That story can still make me emotional.

The last few days were absolutely exhausting for me. I began taking naps on our lunch breaks inside the containers with the corpses. There were approximately 48 bodies per container. I would find one not full and jump into the empty shelf in the cool darkness of the refrigerated container and sleep for an hour or more. It was heaven for a short time each day. I wore a mask that blocked the smell completely, and I would dream of New Zealand—not my house, but beaches and the sea and forests where I used to camp. It was so nice, until one day my boss found me and looked quite shocked and concerned for me, sleeping among the dead.

He asked me to go back to Bangkok for a few days, but I refused. I couldn't leave now. He actually asked me many times to go back, and I often wondered why. I didn't know until months later, when we all met up again in Bangkok, that most people worked for only two or three days and then went home for a few days, so they didn't burn out. I just assumed they were out in the field for a few days, and then came back. It hadn't occurred to me that only the bosses and I worked for a solid two weeks without a break!

The bodies finally did stop coming in. We knew there were plenty more out there, but they were now hard to find. Either they had been taken out to sea, or were buried in the rubble. And so my day came to leave Bang Muang. I was torn between staying and continuing my work at Watt Yan Yao temple, or having to face the fact that I could lose my job in Chon Buri. My visa update was overdue, so getting deported with a fine was a possibility. The work was nearing completion and most of the others on my team had already gone.

So after just a few good-byes, I left very early in the morning. I knew I would see my brothers again in the near future; a good-bye was unnecessary here and now. I hitched a nice ride in a pickup to Phuket. It was so nice to lay in the back, alone on a hard plastic floor, and not smell the dead.

My story ends with a trip back on an air force cargo plane. I saw some fresh volunteers get off my plane and thought how lucky they were that they hadn't been here when it started. I felt like a veteran compared to them. They looked eager and excited; I looked like shit.

Since then I have never stopped working to help the dead and the living. I can't stop.

Go with the Flow, Adapt to the Changes

≈

Ronda M. Faciane, RN, BSN

I REMEMBER GROWING UP in New Orleans, listening intently as the old folks would chronicle how residents survived the 1965 hurricane named Betsy. These were the stories of dire straits and heroism, but to me they seemed a fancifully spun yarn, almost fictitious. Throughout the subsequent years, New Orleans experienced many a hurricane threat, always being spared by a last-minute turn of fate that seemed to steer the storms away and spare the city. We became quite accustomed to our good fortune, always counting on our prayers being answered and saving us from the ravages of another Betsy. But on August 29, 2005, our luck tragically came to an end. This is my account of Hurricane Katrina and its aftermath, depicting the human desire to be spared disaster and to find shelter against the unpredictability of nature.

Watching an approaching hurricane and its path is almost ritualistic in its effect on the observer. The constant reports and warnings by the local and state governments to take no unnecessary risks preceding the storm are unsettling, causing an uneasiness in one's mind as to what is about to happen. I knew that I would be staying in the city during the storm, as I am a registered nurse, employed by the Veterans Administration Hospital located in downtown New Orleans. All essential personnel and first responders such as the police, fire and rescue, medical, and city government were required to stay and assist with emergencies and patients. With my immediate family evacuated west to the city of Lafayette, I felt at ease, not knowing the ordeal I was about to face.

As I reported to the hospital that Sunday morning, I was met by my friend and coworker, Christine. We are both operating room nurses. We assumed our duties would consist of being available for emergency surgeries and to assist where needed. Now, anyone who has ever worked in an operating room knows that a different procedural environment and knowledge base exist here compared to other medical arenas. There are more specialized practices involved in working in an OR, which render us of little use to the rest of the nursing world. As luck (or the lack thereof) would have it, though, we were immediately asked to report to the wards to assist with basic nursing care.

The nurses there had been working 16 hours or more and needed immediate relief. I took a deep breath and said to myself, "Ronda, you have to go with the flow, adapt to the changes, and you will be fine." Suddenly, as if out of some bad dream, I found myself in charge of a team of 15 patients, charting, basic care, and my Achilles' heel: the computerized administration of medications. These are daunting tasks for an OR nurse. But nursing is like riding a bicycle—only this time I needed training wheels, which were nowhere to be found.

"Sink or swim!" I told myself, as I laughed about my predicament to stave off the nerves. I eventually balanced myself and, through a series of adaptations, managed to do my best and work safely in a very stressful situation.

In a crisis, with expectations changing constantly, how you adapt to your circumstances and the trust you have in your skill sets will ultimately determine your success or failure. As I finished my shift around 8:00 P.M., I was exhausted. I can't honestly tell you what was more fatigued: my body or my mind. The cafeteria served spaghetti for dinner that first night. We were like schoolchildren on a camping trip, giddy and playful, as we gathered together with coworkers and their families and then retired for the night. None of us would be prepared for the disaster that we would awaken to that next fateful morning.

The wake-up call came about two or three o'clock Monday morning. Over the noise of breaking glass, we could hear instructions being shouted to move the patients to the hallway and away from windows. I can still hear the winds now, a loud rhythmic whipping sound that plays over and again in my mind. The reality of the disaster began setting in, the juvenile playfulness of hours earlier evaporating as I was consumed by patient care and oblivious to the outside events that were unfolding. As I peered momentarily out of a window, I could see the water rising over car tops, and I heard a radio report saying the levees had broken. Four or five feet of water had flooded Central Business District, temporarily shielding my mind from the far worse reality I would face later.

As I worked alongside my colleagues, I could not help but admire their dedication, as many of them had family members yet unaccounted for and who hadn't been heard from for hours. They had homes that were being destroyed, irreplaceable heirlooms, and family treasures washed away by this howling beast that was upon us. It was at this time that I felt a kinship with my coworkers and their family members who were helping with tasks and with the patients. We were all one family, bound together by the compassion we felt for one another and our will to survive. That feeling gave me comfort and faith in my ability to overcome this great challenge.

The electrical grid had given out, and the humid August heat was stifling without air-conditioning. Soon we cut our uniforms to Bermuda-short scrubs and stripped to T-shirts.

I just kept telling myself, "Go with the flow, adapt to the changes."

We did have emergency power and were able to provide fans to the more critical patients. Opening windows in the hospital is a complex operation that requires a special tool. That tool became precious equipment, and it is now part of the standard emergency kit. Eventually, the windows were opened and, with the passing of the storm, a quiet settled over us that did not reflect the tragic flooding and turmoil the rest of the city was experiencing.

Medicine becomes quite rudimentary in a crisis without power. Our role becomes assessment, assessment, and more assessment. Each day offered new challenges, but safe practices were not compromised.

It became advantageous for me to work during the hurricane. As my family sat day after day feeling helpless with constant television images depicting the despair, destruction, and dying in New Orleans, I worked to exhaustion each day, slept during the night, and awoke to repeat the cycle. I remember the staff psychiatrist passing Xanax, an anti-anxiety drug, to the employees, which seemed funny to me at the time. I was totally focused on patient care, almost to the point of being dissociated from outside events. I could not process those other events; it would have been too overwhelming.

The world outside our VA home was absolute chaos. We heard nightmare stories of the Superdome, Convention

Center, and Charity Hospital. But our world remained
calm and quiet. There never arose a feeling that we would
not survive this experience; our patients adapted reason-
ably well.

We worked in the heat with emergency power and no
running water, and the days passed. Everyone awaited our
evacuation with anticipation. How the food service continued I do not know, as it was evident our food and water
resources were dwindling. The Sunday-night spaghetti
dinner seemed ages ago, being replaced on our last day in
the facility with peanut butter and jelly sandwiches, the
old reliable staple for all disaster preparations. Thursday
morning we were told to prepare the patients for evacuation. A few months earlier, the hospital had fitted all
beds with Evacusled equipment, which is considered the
gold standard for patient evacuations. Evacusleds cocoon
the patient with the mattress and roll on 25 underside
wheels. They can be used by a single rescuer and were a
godsend.

Moving the patients down flights of stairs was back-
breaking work, but everyone toiled together to make our
efforts successful. It would be hard to single out one person's contribution over another's, but soon we had everyone at the staging area awaiting evacuation. I take great
pride in being a part of the unit that day, and I am still
amazed by our cooperative effort.

Hours went by before we were evacuated, which
made it very difficult to maintain patient care. Another
nurse and I procured medications for our patients, and I

remembered a silly little thought about accounting for the narcotics. That thought vanished, as I knew the rules had all changed now and we had to adapt our procedures in order to successfully meet the needs of our patients.

"Go with the flow, adapt to the changes." I must have told myself that a thousand times.

We distributed medications for pain, provided food and water, and assisted with basic care needs. It was not until later that evening that two National Guard vehicles arrived, and the ambulatory patients were evacuated first. The disappointment that the remaining patients, the staff, and I felt was almost overwhelming, but we knew we had to hunker down for the evening. We took the more critical patients back to the emergency room and maintained care for the others in the staging area.

It seemed a very long night, one in which we had to endure the pain of seeing some of our patients pass away. This was a crushing blow to the staff. The stress of the day and the loss of lives were beginning to unravel me emotionally. I faded off to sleep on an exam table, hoping for a better day the next morning.

I awoke to the Arkansas National Guard arriving, and the gratitude I felt to our neighboring state and the volunteers who came from there to help us lifted my spirits tremendously. Our VA brothers and sisters—fellow nurses and physicians who came along with each vehicle—moved in to help care for the patients until they could be transferred to another facility. Just as this was happening, reality slapped me in the face, as if it hadn't already. As the vehicle I was in left the loading dock, I remember seeing the Hyatt Regency Hotel, a beautiful glass building, in ruins. This was the city I had lived in all my life, and a part of my history was taken away by this disaster. I was never going to get it back.

As we reached the airport, a helicopter brought a lone little boy with one shoe. I did not see any of his family members anywhere—they had probably been taken by the storm—and the enormity of the disaster brought me to tears that I fought to hold back. It was a most emotionally trying time there at the airport. A sea of patients lay on the floor of the airport, as we passed by people who were begging for help that I could not provide. It was like having a loaf of bread to feed hundreds, a true feeling of utter inadequacy. The magnitude of the situation overwhelmed all emergency services.

I was very proud of the young servicemen and services such as the Job Corps that sent members to assist with medical care in the airport. The VA also separated itself by sending medical staff to assist with patients until they were transported to other VA facilities in the region. Expecting the sort of old-fashioned K rations the military used to provide, we were pleasantly surprised by the MREs (Meals Ready to Eat) and bottled water we received after our arrival. It felt like a five-star dining experience for everyone, MREs having come a long way since the days of the K ration.

After surviving the oppressive humidity and sweltering heat at the hospital, we were in the cold air-conditioning of the airport, a transition that was difficult for many patients. So I commandeered any blankets I could find and gave them to the most critical patients. This, as to be expected, started arguments from the patients who did not receive any blankets. Patience was wearing thin, and we were all emotionally and physically exhausted. The final straw came when only one plane arrived and half of the group had to be left behind. The disappointment was almost equal to being left behind on that Thursday night. I was asked by the chief surgery resident, a friend, to remain with the second group. The patients in our group were angry. I am sure this emotion was an expression of many other emotions that could only express themselves in anger at the time.

"Go with the flow, adapt to the changes." Again this thought crossed my mind. It was at that time I remembered I had Hershey's miniature candies in my bag and began to distribute them to everyone. On this occasion, even the diabetics could indulge in chocolate. It was amazing to me the soothing feeling that overcame the group. So many things were out of our control, but this moment reminded us of other times and strengthened us as a group not to fold against ourselves. Thank you, Mr. Hershey! I am sure you could not have envisioned such a purpose for your product.

The second plane did finally come that evening and we were transported to Little Rock, Arkansas. I always felt it was my destiny to work during the hurricane. I know that the experience has tested and strengthened me as a nurse and as a person. My faith in the kindness of our fellow human beings will forever be reaffirmed by this experience. I say thank you to the many people who have touched my life and the many lives affected by this hurricane. Today, my family often speaks in terms of before or after Katrina, like B.C. and A.D. For me, I think of the strength I gained in the midst of the greatest natural disaster to have taken place in my lifetime.

"Go with the flow, adapt to the changes." That was this nurse's life.

Angels on the Battlefield

~

Rhona Knox Prescott, RN, MSW

I SERVED AS AN army nurse in Vietnam from February 1967 through February 1968. It was a chaotic, trying time, encompassing two infamous TET offensives. (The military campaign was called TET because it began on the first day of the New Year according to the lunar calendar: Tet Nguyen Dan.) TET, and the months just before, were times of enemy buildups and especially high casualties for Americans.

Although nurses were generally assigned to large base areas, because of overwhelming casualties many nurses and medics found themselves in quite primitive places with less than the best protection and minimal equipment. I was sent to Camp Radcliff at An Khe because of my surgical training, field experience, and administrative background. At the time, An Khe was the base camp for the elite First Cavalry Division in what was known as the Central Highlands.

Casualties were especially heavy right then, and the "Cav," as we called them, didn't want to lose specially trained men through the medical evacuation process. So an existing first aid station was converted to a 100-bed surgical hospital. Eight nurses, including myself, the ranking nurse, worked under tents with minimal medical equipment.

Small miracles occurred there every day. Mayonnaise jars became chest drainage bottles. With some crude additions, they also became suction machines. Corpsmen from a previous war taught us all to suture and perform surgeries.

Fortunately, none of us required much sleep, nor did we become ill. We worked continuously for impossible stretches of time to treat as many wounded soldiers as were brought in by helicopter each day. Once I pulled a 36-hour shift; another time we were in surgery so long they put straws under our surgical masks and instructed us to drink highly sweetened Kool-Aid just to keep our blood sugar up so we could keep working.

We had so many surgical patients they were forced to lie on the tent floors to recuperate after surgery. All the cots were full. Supplies and surgical instruments had to be shared. Antibiotics had long ago been used up. Our precious troops were dying for lack of supplies.

And then the angels came.

Two corpsmen—boys, really, hardly grown men—reported to me one morning. They looked more clean-cut than most of the soldiers in Nam, and they each showed more maturity than their ages would warrant. An Khe was one of the least desirable and most challenging duty spots. They had been assigned here as punishment. Well-educated men, they had both just been released from the stockade, where they had been placed for refusing to "hump ammo," or load 200-pound rounds of artillery pieces, after seeing what the results were. It was unclear to me why medics were in an artillery unit in that capacity, but just the same they were.

And now they were here to work for me. They came to An Khe humble and beaten down, but not without integrity.

"We will do anything—absolutely anything—to save lives, Captain. No matter how risky," one said, the other nodding in agreement. They seemed sincere, almost as desperate as I.

I called their bluff.

The only safe way in and out of An Khe was by air, and the flights were few and far between. The road was mined several times daily, and many vehicles had blown up. Needed medical supplies could not be legally obtained, let alone transported in, since our facility was considered only a medical clearing company, intended to provide just minor care. It had not been declared an official hospital—one of the many paperwork snafus of the war.

I briefed them both on the risks of land travel and the desperate need for supplies. With great guilt, fear, and uncommon prayer, I sent these two out to almost certain death, over the road, off the record, and unauthorized, to get supplies however they could.

Five long days went by. I began mentally composing the letters to their families. But angels were with them. They returned with an intact truck loaded with penicillin, surgical instruments, a real suction machine, and even a steel litter on real wheels.

What a moment of faith we felt when they drove in! Many lives were saved because of their effort and grace from on high. And as a result, we all were reenergized to continue our breakneck schedule.

So heroes can come out of stockades, angels do roam the battlefield, and there is a God ... even in war.

The Day of the Great Wave:
The Story of a Young Hero

~

Perry Prince

IT WAS A moment or two before I saw him, pressed against his father's side and so much smaller than the dozen men seated together in this bare cement-block room. We were in the Battialoa grade school, which now provided temporary shelter to the bedraggled members of a ravaged neighboring community.

It was March 2005, and I was part of a team of disaster mental health workers who had come to Sri Lanka to help survivors of the December 2004 Asian tsunami in a small Tamil village on the eastern coast.

A line from a poem I'd learned long ago popped suddenly into my head: *All that was left of them, left of six hundred.* I was newly arrived and in shock myself from the heartbreaking devastation in the area. Here, where there had been a very different kind of battle from the one Tennyson wrote about, only a third of the original population had survived, and loss is what I saw in every face. Loss and terrible, desolate grief.

Before December 27, 2004, 5,000 people had lived in this village, where their parents and grandparents and the many generations before them had also lived. Then, in less than an hour, more than 3,000 men, women, and children disappeared suddenly, violently. How could anyone even comprehend what had happened—this wild, raging force that attacked so suddenly, and departed as quickly, leaving behind a wasteland of destruction and death?

These men had gathered in the schoolroom simply to tell their stories, to describe what had happened to them and their families in an assault more vicious than the worst nightmare that any had ever imagined. The tsunami was a monster larger and far more terrible than the great black serpent in the tale that they had sometimes used to make their children behave.

"Be good," they had told them, "or the great black serpent will get you!"

But no one had ever believed there could be a demon like the one that had destroyed their village and murdered their loved ones without any reason at all.

While the survivors in this group all seemed shrunken by confusion and sadness, their voices were agitated and loud as each competed with the rest to recount his tale of horror. All needed to be heard, but in the excited, over-lapping din, it was impossible to make out coherent words or sentences.

Finally, I reached into my backpack and withdrew the first small, smooth object I touched: a plastic tube of sunscreen, which I offered as a "talking stick," the holder would have the privilege of speaking and also the responsibility for passing the tube to the next speaker when his tale was finished.

To my surprise, after our translator explained the contents of the container, several of the men opened it carefully after speaking and applied a small amount to their right arms. Without intending it, I had begun a group ritual. And when I offered a little joke—that I could perhaps now expect to see them all with a patch of skin the color of mine—I witnessed the first smiles I had seen since my arrival.

After several people told their stories, the pressure to speak lessened. When I asked who would like to be next, everyone began to point excitedly to the only child in the room, a boy I had seen sitting close to his father's side. Although he looked like a slender 8-year-old, I later learned that he was actually 11. The "talking stick" was put into his hands, and after a moment the boy, named Oli, stood and began to speak.

He had been outside playing with other children when the first wave struck. There was a sudden noise, followed by a rush of water advancing from the ocean toward his house. His fisherman father was far out at sea, but his mother, sisters, and aunts were in the house, and Oli ran inside to warn them. At first, the women shrugged him aside, but as water began to enter the house, the whole confused group ran outdoors to find out what was happening.

Already, a larger wave was coming. Oli and his brother climbed a tree, but then he saw that his mother, sisters, and the family dog had been pulled out into the nearby lagoon, and he clambered down to start searching for them.

As he described the scene, how they and their neighbors were swept into the lagoon, along with cooking stoves, tables, chairs, outriggers, and canoes, Oli's voice became more urgent. His small hands clutching the sunscreen talking stick, he described how some managed to pull themselves out of the lagoon and back onto the sandy soil, only to be struck by a third, much larger wave. Swept once more into the lagoon, they were assaulted by flying debris, more damaged and broken boats, and parts of houses ripped apart by the wave.

Oli worked and fished with his father. He was a strong swimmer and experienced with boats. When he saw a canoe that was still upright, he pulled himself into it to continue the search for his family. Because girls and women are not taught to swim in this area of Sri Lanka, he knew he had very little time.

Relieved to soon find his mother and one of his sisters clinging to pieces of wood, he managed to pull them into the canoe before another wave tipped it over. His mother disappeared instantly, but Oli somehow got his sister back to land and lifted her into a tree.

He discovered another usable boat and he tried once more to find his mother. When he realized that there was no longer hope of saving her, he worked frantically to rescue anyone he could. Then another wave came, capsizing the boat and uprooting the tree that held his sister, who instantly disappeared from sight.

Out in the open ocean, where Oli's father was fishing, there was no indication of trouble on land. He had no idea what was happening at home until he returned in the late afternoon and discovered that the entire village had disappeared and more than 30 members of his family had perished, leaving Oli and himself as the sole survivors.

The boy finished his story, handed the talking stick to a man sitting nearby, and took his place once more at his father's side. More stories were told in low and sorrowful voices, until, at last, a great sigh went through the group and all was silent.

Quietly, the men got up and filed out, leaving our translator, Gunalan, my fellow worker, Tom, and myself in the bare room. The talking stick had been placed carefully in the center of the floor. As I put it in my backpack, although it contained a lot less sunscreen than at the beginning of the meeting, it felt much heavier in my hand.

In the weeks that followed, I saw Oli many times, sometimes with his father but never with other children.

His heroism had strangely isolated him, a child who was no longer a child, in a changed and saddened world.

Clowns to the Rescue

~

Dionetta Hudzinski, RN, MN

I AM A NURSE who works primarily with people in pain and people who are dying. So it was not surprising that I found myself leaving my home in Marston Mills, Massachusetts, and heading off to Ground Zero in New York City one year after the World Trade Center tragedy. What was surprising was that I was doing it as a clown. Now this might seem irreverent to some and shocking to others, but I must tell you it was one of the most awesome experiences of my life.

First, I must share some background information. I have been a professional nurse since 1969 and a professional clown since 1995. My clowning is a gift, a legacy, given to me by one of my hospice patients. Bob Bennett was a Shriner Clown and he was dying of cancer. I was called in to help control his pain. Twenty-four hours later, Bob was essentially pain-free and ready to live what was left of his life. One of his last wishes was to form a clown alley, a group of people interested in clowning, and pass on his art of clowning to others. I had used this gift as a way to reach out to people in hospitals and nursing homes, and then in New York City, to lift people's spirits and help heal their wounded hearts.

I was part of a group of about 18 clowns from all over the United States who gathered in New York City to bring hope and laughter as New Yorkers faced the anniversary of the 9/11 tragedy. Some of these same clowns ministered to the rescue workers during the weeks and months following 9/11.

Instead of being told to go away, to mind our own business, we were invited to clown around and bring a welcomed respite to the sadness that surrounded the area that once was the Twin Towers. We passed out over 1,000 red noses, seeds of hope (baggies of fruit loops), and clown stickers. We visited every police station and fire station that had been affected that fateful day. We listened to the stories that were told of where they were, the loved ones who were lost, what they felt, and what they've done since then.

We rode the buses and subways and walked the streets of New York City in full clown makeup and costume. I had been to New York City several times before, as I grew up in upstate New York. But the city was somehow different then. There was tenderness and a vulnerability to it.

The people did not ignore us; they talked to us. Strangers on the street walked up to us and talked to us, the clowns. They shared their stories and their fears, and they even cried with us. Some told us they had not talked about this to anyone, but here they were on the street talking to strange-looking creatures, the clowns. I felt privileged to be a part of this moment.

One particular story sticks with me even today. We were at one of the fire stations when the crew was just returning from a call. As they gathered around us, I was drawn to a young firefighter named John. I asked him where he was on 9/11. He was home, as it was his day off. As soon as he heard the call to go out, he rushed to the towers to help—but by the time he arrived, there was no one to save. Every one of the crew from his station who was on duty that day died. John told me he really did not know whether he still wanted to be a firefighter, let alone whether he still wanted to live.

We talked for some time. We hugged and we cried. Suddenly, he pointed to a pin I had on my costume that read "I'm in charge of Diddly-Squat" and said, "That's how I feel." So I undid the pin and pinned it onto John's suspenders. Later, one of the other firefighters asked John what he had on his suspenders, and he said, "I'm in charge of Diddly-Squat, and that," he pointed to me, "is Diddly-Squat."

Later that week, as the world watched and as the first-anniversary memorial services took place, reporters interviewed many of the firefighters. One of those firefighters was my John. And I will never forget what he said: "The clowns came and they saved my life."

I still get goose bumps thinking about it.

I now have a new clown character named Diddly-Squat in honor of John and the power that the clown has to touch lives in a very special way. We as nurses have that same power to touch lives and to heal the hurt. Clowning is just another therapeutic tool in our vast array of tools and techniques we can use when caring for our patients.

Trauma, Healing, and Serendipity in the Sichuan Province, China

~

Elaine Miller-Karas, LCSW

ON MAY 12, 2008, a massive earthquake hit the Sichuan Province of China. Tens of thousands of people died, thousands were injured, and millions were left homeless. This catastrophic world event became more personal when our nonprofit agency, the Trauma Resource Institute (TRI), was invited to bring our innovative trauma treatment, the Trauma Resiliency Model (TRM), to the Chinese people in the Sichuan Province.

TRI was cofounded in 2007 by Dr. Laurie Leitch and me. Our mission is to provide education about the treatment of traumatic stress and build sustainability projects by training community leaders, doctors, teachers, nurses, and counselors in areas hard-hit by disaster. We have worked in Thailand, Africa, the United States, and China.

We now coordinate a Chinese Earthquake Relief Project (CHERP) along with a nonprofit arm of Chindex, a Chinese corporation. The project is cosponsored by the World Health Organization.

We were witness to horrific stories of death and despair, but we also saw the remarkable resilience and optimism of the Chinese people as they slowly rebuilt their communities after this devastating natural disaster. This is a recounting of our work in the field after the Sichuan earthquake, with our team of psychotherapists, trainers, and translators.

Each day, we gather for the hour or so ride in an old ambulance that has seen better days for the trip from Mianyang to Beichuan. There are no seat belts. We sit on tiny plastic seats and hold on tightly to old IV straps hanging from the ceiling. The seats are hard, but the conversations lively. At times we sing songs from the 60s or from our favorite Broadway shows. It is warm and humid, and the smoke from our driver's cigarettes permeates the air. Rita, Harriet, and Rhine, our translators, sing Chinese songs. They giggle and we are touched by the rhythmic sounds of their sweet, clear voices.

As we ride through the roads toward Beichuan, we are confronted with the ruins of the damaged buildings. We understand much has been cleared away, but there is enormous damage. It will take months, or years, to remove the debris.

There are also the vistas of new life. The crimson red of the bricks of rebuilding threads through the roadside alongside the blue tents of recovery. The color yellow splashes the landscape of the roadsides, as corncobs hang to dry in front of the blue tents. The roadways are full of life, children laughing and playing, people talking, riding their scooters and bicycles, and building new homes.

Yet as we drive closer to Beichuan Hospital, the mood changes within the ambulance as the damage from the earthquake becomes more vivid, more global. The carcasses of ruined buildings flood us. There is pallor in the air, the day smoky from the fires of rebuilding. The mountains loom, surrounding the ruins, and frame the damage, making the images more discrete.

We arrive at the hospital and are guided to a medium-size room, full of computers and two or three people working. A public health officer greets us. They tell us that most of the medical personnel are taking a mandatory exam today and only a few people will be available to teach.

The room slowly fills with doctors and nurses. The noise from the building distorts our voices as we try to speak. There is the sound of a chain saw, then a bullhorn, and over a short period of time five or six cell phones blast through the room. The room is like a tin can, and each time someone moves a chair or steps outside, the sounds of movement vibrate and ricochet off the walls.

The translators have difficulty hearing us through the commotion.

The participants are clearly in a high state of activation, a term we use to describe symptoms of hyperarousal that can include agitation, anxiety, hypervigilance, irritability, and, in extreme cases, anger. At the resettlement village, we see anxiety, agitation, and irritability. The staff is shorthanded because of the exam. Also, half of the healthcare providers were killed in the earthquake. Because of the activation of the doctors and nurses, we decide to shorten the training and spend the second part of the day providing sessions for them. Flexibility and change are as important as the air we breathe when we are in a disaster area.

Later in the day, before we return to Mianyang and to our hotel, Dr. Zhau, our host in the field, takes us to the vista site, high on a mountaintop, to see the City of Beichuan. It lies in the smoky mist, half buried by the looming mountains that destroyed it in one giant movement of the earth. Now it is a shrine: people from all over China come to pay homage to the dead.

The Chinese government put a huge barbed-wire fence around the parameters of the city, which is down in a valley. The fence can be seen for miles. Local residents have set up food stands and concessions selling incense and photos from the destruction.

It is the most sobering vista I have ever experienced. Cars drive up and citizens quietly leave their cars and, with a solemn reverence, look out into the valley that is now a tomb for literally thousands upon thousands of people. We are silent and many of us have tears in our eyes. The enormity of the loss is omnipresent.

Next, we visit the ruins of Biechuan Middle School, where 2,000 children and teachers lost their lives. There is a skeleton of two stories of what was a five-story building and a pile of rubble that runs wide and high. Within the rubble, vestiges of happier times are visible—school desks, notebooks, and probably the saddest of all: children's shoes strewn throughout.

Parents of the dead children have left flowers, bowls of fruit, poems, and colorful umbrellas at the site in memory of their children. We stand on the basketball court, which was unscathed. Our team of 12 stares in silence, transfixed by the rubble and the loss. Our young translators are overcome with grief. Those of us from America stand next to them with our arms around them as they shed tears for the innocence and the lost potential of each one of those little lives that will never grow up, who will be encased in this cement tomb for eternity.

As we stand here in our grief, we are suddenly reminded of the resilience of life when we hear the sound of children laughing. Their voices echo through the school site as they play on a nearby hillside.

When we arrive back at the hotel, we hold our team meeting. The next morning, we will visit the resettlement camp. We are exhausted. We embrace and plan our starting time for the next day, then retreat to our rooms for respite and reflection.

We have learned to have a plan, but not to be tied to any plan because arrival at our destination may present us with a different challenge. Our team members work well together, and we have developed a nice collaboration with our translators. The shared experience and our attention to the group process have created a strong bond among the 12 of us.

When we arrive at the resettlement camp, we are escorted to a large community room. Bookshelves of children's books line one wall. There are desks at one end, and many chairs in front of the desks. An elderly woman, 72 years of age, arrives first. She tells us how she and her husband survived the earthquake and that the land for the resettlement camp used to be where her home stood. She is very talkative and tells us she is doing fine since the earthquake. She is glad to be alive when so many have lost their lives.

Within a few minutes, the room fills with adults and children. There are about 40 people in the room and there is the rustling of anticipation. Children are laughing and crying. They wait for us to speak.

We begin by talking to the group about who we are and why we have come. I relate a story about being in many earthquakes in California and how unsettling it is after—still feeling like the earth is shaking when it isn't and feeling shaky in my legs. The people respond to this personal experience, and when I ask if anyone has had an experience like mine, the whole room practically stands up and shouts in agreement.

We share that we are going to show them some simple skills that might help them feel better. Then we introduce TRM's grounding skill. Grounding helps orient a person to their own body in relationship to present time and space by bringing the person's awareness to how their body is supported by the chair they sit in, how their feet contact the ground, and where they are in relationship to the room they are in. Grounding gives them a sense of relationship to the earth, time and space, and is necessary to sustain authentic presence and to experience physical, emotional, and spiritual safety. The exercise is simple. Many people respond that they feel their breathing slowing down.

One woman raises her hand and says she felt her heart rate go up when she pushed her feet into the ground. I ask her for permission to work with her. She agrees and we begin to work together. I introduce the TRM treatment. Soon after, each team member is working in a corner of the room. Friends and family surround the family member we are working with to give added support. There is also a great deal of curiosity.

The woman says that her legs have jerked and shaken uncontrollably since the earthquake. She had been pinned in the rubble of her home, her toes crushed, and had been amputated. Afterward, she spent many weeks in the hospital. Today, she reports insomnia as well as the inability to control the movements in her legs.

The TRM skills were introduced to her over the next hour. During the course of the treatment, she indicates that she feels a sense of inner peace that she has not felt since the earthquake. An image was awakened within her that she thinks she can use to help calm her body and mind. She replicates the posture for us. She shares with us that she will place herself in the position with her one hand on her heart and one on her stomach when she goes to bed. She thinks this will help her sleep better and maybe remove the images from her head.

As she is reflecting on this new thought and showing us the posture, we invite her to sense her whole body and to notice the changes she has experienced since we started. As we end the session, the woman smiles. She appears more peaceful. She reports her heart rate is in normal range and her breathing even. We can all see that her leg has stopped shaking.

After the session, the woman insists that I come to see her home in the resettlement camp. We walk with her and a band of children, who dance around us with happy smiles and gestures that indicate they want their photos taken.

Her home is two simple rooms, one a kitchen and sitting area and the other a sleeping room. She brings fresh peanuts for us to eat, then asks me about my life. I share photos of my children. It is such a sweet moment of sharing between two women across cultures. As I leave, we embrace. She insists I take a bag full of peanuts. A heartfelt thank-you is exchanged by both of us.

The people of Sichuan Province are very proud of their unique, flavorful food that is full of colorful vegetables, spices, and richness. After our training days, our hosts end our day by taking us to a festive restaurant. They thank us profusely with customary toasts with small glasses of beer, held in a certain way to express their respect to us.

On this day, our ambulance pulls up to a lone building, a restaurant serving "hot pot." It is one of the only buildings still standing amid the earthquake rubble. Our entourage, which now includes some of our hosts from the city, is seated at two large tables, each with a hot pot in the center. As we enter the restaurant, I recognize a family from earlier in the week. I worked with their son, a 15-year-old, who had survived the Beichuan Middle School collapse. They rush toward me and, with the help of my translator, tell me that since the treatment, their son has slept through the night and is no longer having frequent flashbacks from the day of the earthquake. They each take my hand and shake it vigorously. I am touched deeply by the expression of gratitude and struck by the serendipity of the family eating at the same restaurant. My eyes well up as they take my hands into theirs. Although my translator helps with their words, there is a deeper exchange between us that speaks through the language of our eyes. A deep place in my heart and soul tenderly rocks as the mother recounts her son's improvement. This story will keep me going during the times that I despair, wondering why on earth I have traveled so far away from the comforts and safety of my home in California.

One of the physicians who is traveling with our project tells me as I sit down after I exchange good-byes with the family that it may not have been serendipity. Rather, it may have been that the parents sought out where the "foreign experts" would lunch, so as to pay their respects to me. Serendipity or not, the exchange is one I will never forget.

Working and training in the Sichuan Province has been a full, textured experience, as rich and flavorful as the food of this region. I have been struck by the resilience of the Chinese people and their tenacity to rebuild. I have been touched by the laughter and playfulness of the children and the courage of the people who bring their tender tragedies to the "foreign experts," as they call us, to try to alleviate their suffering and pain.

Our treatment approach is not bound by Western traditional psychotherapy, but by an understanding of cutting-edge research about the brain and an awareness of our shared experience of being human. It is about how tragedy strikes us all in a similar way in our body and mind, whether we grew up in China or the United States. As we understand the wisdom of the healing potential within the body and mind, our worlds merge. Although we come from different places on the globe, respectful of cultural differences, we are connected in profound ways.

Miracle at Landing Zone Ross

≈

Robert B. Robeson

"I think I should say one word, too, a special word, about the 'Dust Offs'—the medevacs. This was a great group of men. All those who flew them, all those who did it. Courage above and beyond the call of duty was sort of routine to them. It was a daily thing, part of the way they lived. That's the great part, and it meant so much to every last man who served there. Whether he ever got hurt or not, he knew Dust Off was there."
—Gen. Creighton W. Abrams Jr.,
Army Chief of Staff at AAAA Honors
Luncheon, Sheraton Park Hotel,
Washington, D.C., October 13, 1972

THE RECOLLECTION OF that unbelievable medical evacuation mission on Saturday, September 13, 1969—two days prior to my 27th birthday—flashed through my mind. I was standing bareheaded at attention under a scorching early afternoon sun in Da Nang, South Vietnam, in our unit area on the shore of scenic Da Nang Harbor. It was mid-March 1970. The aide for Col. D. W. Pratt, the U.S. Army 95th Evacuation Hospital commander, was reading my citation for a Distinguished Flying Cross, which our entire "Dust Off" crew had received.

The memory alone of the danger and drama surrounding that mission was enough to make me sweat even more than I already was. I'd been in the country barely two months at that time, but had already seen more of war at 26 years of age than I had ever cared to imagine. As John Keats so aptly stated, "Nothing ever becomes real till it is experienced."

That's part of the reason why Chief Warrant Officer 2 John Ball would mean so much to me. John was 32 years of age and had four children. This former marine turned army aviator was an old soldier of many military campaigns around the planet.

As operations officer for the 236th Medical Detachment (Helicopter Ambulance), headquartered at Red Beach, I'd scheduled myself to spend five days, September 10–14, as John's copilot. He was an aircraft commander and also one of our instructor pilots. We'd be stationed at our field site aid station at Landing Zone (LZ) Baldy, located approximately 25 miles south of Da Nang. We gathered the rest of our crew—a medic and crew chief—and flew out to cover action that would keep us in the air over 31 hours, which included 12½ night hours, evacuating dead and wounded.

On September 11, our supported infantry units were hit hard by the North Vietnamese Army. We were airborne 11 hours that day and 10 hours on the 12th. We'd slide out of the sky on mission after mission, picking up torn and broken bodies.

We'd already flown over three hours before the sun came up on September 13, and had finally shut down to snatch a few z's. About midmorning another mission was called in. We quickly scrambled after only a momentary rest. We were in the air, returning from this mission with a load of patients, when a second urgent request was broadcast over our FM radio. It was another "insecure" landing zone reportedly under heavy enemy fire. While I called for UH-1C helicopter gunship support from the "Firebirds," who also flew out of Baldy, John landed and unloaded these patients. Then he lifted off again in the direction of four Americans who had been seriously wounded by small arms fire.

Between air-to-air and air-to-ground communications, I said my usual silent prayer for our safety and the safety of our patients.

As we approached the area of contact a few "klicks" (kilometers) southwest of LZ Center—a towering artillery base jutting nearly straight up hundreds of feet above the surrounding terrain—concentrated artillery fire could be seen bracketing a heavily wooded area. This was soon cut off so our two gunships could make gun runs on enemy positions before we went in. After their second pass, I called for smoke to mark where the ground troops wanted us to land.

Then John bottomed the collective control with his left hand, which governs the pitch of the blades, as we transitioned into a smooth 4,000-feet-per-minute descent. As we fell out of the sky, John reminded me to stay close to my controls, something he'd never mentioned before. John always flew with the force trim on.

The force trim was controlled by an on/off switch, located at the top of the pedestal between both pilots (where our four radios were housed), beneath the instrument panel in front of us. With this switch on, there was an artificial feel or force applied to the cyclic stick—the steering wheel of a helicopter—that held the cyclic in one position. You could manually move the cyclic against this force but, if you released pressure, the cyclic stick would return to its last trimmed position. There was an intermittent force trim release button on the cyclic stick grip that, if depressed and held, released the force trim pressure. John trimmed the aircraft—through the use of this button on the cyclic stick—so that there was rearward pressure on the cyclic at all times. That way the nose of our bird would automatically rise should he be wounded or his hand came off the cyclic stick.

Personally, I never flew with the force trim on because it caused me to lose my "touch" on the cyclic when doing many combat maneuvers. But because John chose to do so, we'd all soon benefit from a special message that would manifest itself directly to my heart.

As we continued a rapid descent and began our approach to the landing zone from the west, "Willie Peter"— (white phosphorous) rockets that had been fired ahead of us by our gunships— suddenly obscured the red smoke from the grenade the ground troops had thrown out.

John grabbed a bunch of pitch with the collective in his left hand and began a tight, 360-degree cyclic climb to his left. With the "bad guys" reported to be so close to the wounded, making the ultimate misjudgment of landing in the wrong area could have been disastrous. "Tango 2-4, this is Dusty," I broadcast over our FM radio. "We lost your smoke because of the Willie Pete. If you could pop one more, we'll attempt another approach. Over."

"Negative on the smoke, Dusty. We're all out down here."

"Okay, we'll drop our own smoke," John said.

With 2-4 visually guiding us, we barreled in on two runs 50 feet above the landing zone tree line as our crew chief dropped smoke grenades under heavy enemy fire. On the second pass, we finally hit our target. Then John circled back to land.

It was because the landing zone was so tight (we couldn't turn around to go out the way we'd come in for fear of hitting someone or something with our tail rotor) that John made the decision he did.

"I'm going up and over to get out of here, Bob," John said over the intercom.

As we topped the trees that hid the enemy force, at about 75 feet, AK-47 (Soviet assault rifles used by the NVA) and other automatic weapons hosed us down from beneath and to both sides of the aircraft. From that split second of time, for the next minute or so, everything seemed to occur in super-slow motion.

"My God, we're going to crash!" John suddenly yelled into his mike. "My cyclic's been shot away!"

Immediately I looked over to see him sweeping his cyclic stick in wide circles around the cockpit—movements that should have made the aircraft spin in circles. But our bird didn't respond. As the Huey's nose began a dive toward the trees, I instinctively reached for my set of controls.

"I've got it," I said.

This is it, I distinctly remember thinking, as enemy rounds continued ventilating our bird. *Today is the day I'm going to die!*

Suddenly the shooting ceased. We'd flown out of the enemy's field of fire.

When I grasped my cyclic, it was immediately evident that force trim pressure no longer existed. The switch was on, but it had zero effect. An inner whisper that I believe came from God impressed me to be *extremely* careful and not move my cyclic more than necessary to stay out of the tops of the trees that our skids were now brushing. I gently eased the cyclic toward me and we began a shallow ascent.

At that moment, the red rpm warning light on the instrument panel illuminated, accompanied by gut-wrenching shrieks in our flight helmets from the low-rpm audio warning. In rapid succession, the yellow master caution light at the top of the instrument panel was next to make its appearance. Glancing down at the emergency panel on the pedestal between us, I saw that the "engine oil" light was illuminated.

Dust Off pilots set normal engine rpm for our operations between 6,400 and 6,600. Ours had bled off to nearly 5,800 in seconds. I knew that if something didn't happen in a hurry, our bird would soon have more characteristics of a crowbar than a crow.

We'd obviously been hit in the engine and oil lines, among other places. Although John had been grazed in his left leg by a round, he immediately reached over to the pedestal and placed the governor switch into the "emergency" position. This provided enough extra engine power to momentarily remain airborne while we discussed our limited options.

We both realized that our engine was losing a lot of oil and could instantaneously seize. If it did, I'd have to auto rotate (descending on the energy in the blades alone, rather than the engine, to make a forced landing). This would mean I'd also have to make a dramatic movement with my cyclic stick at the bottom to flare and dissipate airspeed before touchdown, even if I found an open area. Otherwise, I'd have to make a tree landing.

"What do you want me to do?" I asked John, as I slowly eased in pitch with my left hand, inched up to 500 feet AGL (above ground level), and attained a comfortable 80 knots of indicated airspeed.

"Just keep us in the air," he answered quietly. "Just fly. Maybe we can find a place to put it down where we won't hurt ourselves."

If our engine failed, I wanted to make a running landing. LZ Ross lay straight ahead, 6 miles northwest of LZ Center and 11 miles southwest of LZ Baldy. Ross was located in relatively flat terrain and had a large open area where we often picked up patients. But this was still four to five minutes away.

"I'm gonna shoot for Ross."

"Okay," John said. "I'll call Da Nang and have them get another bird out there to pick us up."

"Sir," SP5 Bill Bergman—our crew chief—broke in on the intercom, "we got our guns at four o'clock high. Looks like they're following us in."

John alerted the Firebirds to our dilemma, and one of them edged close enough under our blades to confirm that we were leaking oil all over the sky.

I did some silent praying en route too. Having been raised as a preacher's kid gave me a wealth of appreciation and insight for this spiritual involvement. I thanked God for allowing us to reach our four patients and for getting all of us out of that miserable landing zone in one piece. Then I asked Him, if it was His will, to help me keep the rest of the pieces intact until we reached LZ Ross.

I bounced our skids a couple of times on the uneven ground at LZ Ross in a short running landing. And when the ground run stopped, *so did our Lycoming jet engine.* All 1,100 "horses" expired at once. Simultaneously, John and I turned to look at each other. Neither of us said a word. We both realized what had just happened.

We transferred our patients and medic to one of the Firebird gunships, and they both lifted off for the aid station at Baldy.

Then John and I did a postflight inspection. We confirmed that all of the engine oil was gone. The last of it formed two small pools in the red clay beneath the aircraft.

It was hours later before we knew "the rest of the story," as broadcaster Paul Harvey would say. After our maintenance crew arrived and sling-loaded (retrieving the aircraft by hoisting it out beneath a large Chinook helicopter through the use of a sling) the bird back to Red Beach in Da Nang, one of them took me aside. He told me he'd reached up and merely *touched* my cyclic stick. It had broken off in his hand.

After removing the metal floor paneling and taking apart the control, he discovered that only a sliver of metal had been holding it in place. That's why I couldn't feel any force trim pressure against my hand. One of the bursts of automatic weapon fire from John's side of the aircraft had completely severed his cyclic stick and had continued its flight beneath our floor panels to nearly take mine with it.

That soft, inner voice had been right on target. To this day, I firmly believe God, or one of His guardian angels, warned me not to move my cyclic any more than necessary and kept our wounded bird flying for over five minutes with little or no oil in the engine.

Simply stated, it was a *miracle*. This is the only explanation that suffices for what happened so long ago.

The campfire of this combat experience has dwindled to crimson coals. I'm 66 years of age, but I often recall details of those precarious moments on that mission (and the 986 other medevac missions in one year for 2,533 patients from both sides of the action). What I discovered—after having seven helicopters shot up by enemy fire and being shot down twice—was that in this kind of rescue work, you never know whose life you will step into or who will step into yours. Additionally, I realized that a growth of character is possible through life-and-death struggles and in taking risks for others. It's always appropriate to help someone who's a little more lost and hurting than we are, because hope and love are what keep humanity going. And that's what rescue work has always been about—even in a combat zone.

Walking Hand in Hand
with Clara Barton

~

Renee Berke, RN

"HURRICANE FLOYD HAS dealt a devastating blow
to North Carolina and they need nurses. Will you be able
to leave in 24 hours?" I took a deep breath. This was what
I had been waiting for, my first national assignment as a
Red Cross disaster nurse. Now, at 71 years of age, I wondered if I could meet the challenge.

A fellow nurse and I accepted the two-week appoint-
ment and, as luck would have it, we didn't have to leave
for three days. This gave us adequate time to buy boots,
pack, notify our friends and families, and otherwise prepare. After arriving in Raleigh, North Carolina, just in

time for a soaking rain, my friend and I were assigned to a hotel.

The next day, we attended an orientation session at the Red Cross headquarters in Smithfield. We were advised to drink only bottled water when we were away from the hotels and to use an antibacterial solution on our hands. We were also told to watch for alligators, poisonous snakes, and red ants. The homes of these creatures had been disturbed because of the hurricane and the resulting floods, and they were angry and more dangerous than usual. I did see a snake in my travels, but my curiosity wasn't piqued. I didn't stay long enough to realize its toxic potential.

Shortly after the orientation, the other nurse and I were separated. She was assigned to a service center in Wilmington and I was sent to Whiteville. The service center I worked in processed hundreds of people who came to express their grief and arrange for the replacement of glasses, medications, dentures, and other necessities and possessions lost or damaged in the flood.

The work days were long, 10 to 12 hours. A strange phenomenon takes place when you are working in unfamiliar surroundings, performing new tasks with people you haven't met before. You find you have taken a step out of your "real life" and begin losing your perception of time. To compensate for this, each service center posts a large sign with the day and date on the wall. I also spent many days in the outreach program going into the flooded areas where the water had receded enough to assess the health needs of the victims. Some roads were still closed because of the residual water and mud. Traveling along the rural areas, we came across workers lifting dead hogs onto a large truck. The stench from the rotting carcasses and polluted water was nauseating.

Some homes were all but demolished. The water had lifted the floorboards so that we had to walk on top of the waves made by the warped floors. Some people were ill from drinking contaminated well water.

As we approached one house, a man who was sitting dejectedly in a rocking chair on a partially collapsed front porch brightened up and waved us into his home. We stood silently as we viewed a house that had been completely destroyed by an overflowing pond that stood next to it. The furniture was sopping wet and the cupboards were water-stained and peeling. Family pictures covered the walls and, miraculously, had remained intact.

The man's wife was ill, so he was caring for their four children. The entire family was infected with scabies and was undergoing treatment at the local hospital. While we were there, a daughter arrived with her boyfriend. She greeted us perfunctorily and, staring into space, sank into a wet sofa.

The father clearly was the strength of the family. He told us they would be all right because he was going to get help from the Red Cross, FEMA, and relatives and friends, which would allow him to return to work.

That evening, while giving my report, I broke down and cried. The courage of the people who had lost so much touched me in a way I will never forget. Twenty-five years ago, when I graduated from college and received my nursing degree, I never dreamed my life would go in this direction. I became a nurse practitioner (NP) and expected to be involved in that area of nursing for many years. But Clara Barton, founder of the American Red Cross, has always been my heroine, and now I felt I was walking hand in hand with her, at least for a little while.

After our two weeks traveling throughout North Carolina, I returned home to Cape Cod on a clear, sunny day. I stepped off the plane with a divided heart: half-steeped in sorrow for the people of North Carolina whose lives took a negative turn and half-filled with joy to be back to my beloved Cape Cod once more.

Beauty and Grace

~

Grace Muthumbi

Wʜᴇɴ ɪ ᴡᴀs 25 years old, I was in an accident that changed my life forever. It taught me what it is to suffer, what it feels like to be abandoned; but it was also transformative, a catalyst for an unexpected metamorphosis that left me all the more beautiful, though this irony did not seem possible at the time.

I was born in Kenya's Central Province to a family of eight children, four boys and four girls. At the time of the accident, I was out of college, living alone, and engaged to be married. The day was like any other day. I came home from the field and lit the burner on the stove. It was a charcoal burner, which is open and emits carbon monoxide as it burns. I started to feel dizzy, my body heavy, and then nothing.

I woke up six hours later, confused and with a splitting headache. The carbon monoxide had knocked me unconscious, and my face had fallen onto the open burner. My face and head had been scalded, my skin burned raw.

I was sent to two nearby district hospitals, but I needed more advanced care. I was finally referred to Kenyatta Hospital in Nairobi, but the doctors and nurses there were on strike, so I did not receive the immediate care that I needed. As a result, terrible scars from the burns masked part of my face and head. I would never look the same again.

My fiancé left me shortly after, disappearing out of my life completely. My friends were no better. I felt discarded, alone, and badly, badly hurt.

I soon closed off from everyone around me. I didn't want anything to do with anyone. I didn't want to act happy. I didn't want anything. I had so many emotions running through me. I cried when I was home, cried when I was out. I just needed someone to listen to me, to show me that I would find acceptance after the accident.

A friend from college, Martha Kihara, did just that. Though not the most talkative, Martha knows when to speak and when to keep quiet. She listened to me for hours. I talked and talked and cried and cried and Martha just listened. After not seeing me for a while, Martha would come by to see how I was doing. Even though she couldn't understand what I was going through, she gave me strength to work through my grief because she stuck by me at a time when few in my life did.

My older sister also gave me strength to cope with what life had dealt me. When I was released from the hospital, I could not be alone because of the emotional state I was in, so my sister took me in. She stayed by my side, counseling me every day to appreciate that I was alive. I was so lucky to have these two women who gave me unconditional support when everyone else abandoned me.

It was through the heartbreak—and my overcoming it—that I found my inspiration to do the kind of work I do today. I learned what it is like to feel isolated, hurt, and alone, but also what it feels like to have someone there for you when it seems as if the world has turned its back on you. That accident and all the issues that followed completely changed me, shifting my thinking from what I had gone through to what others are facing and how I could help. I knew that I had to give back, offer support to people who felt rejected, much like Martha and my sister had for me.

In 2000, I found my calling by accident at a refugee camp where I was introduced to the International Medical Corps (IMC). A relief and development organization, IMC had been working in Kenya for two years, providing medical care and training to the local population. They had other similar programs throughout Africa and soon hired me to work with them in South Sudan.

Sudan is where I was introduced to working with HIV/AIDS. While the program focus was to treat African sleeping sickness, those with HIV needed special care, as their weakened immune systems could do very little against the disease that attacks the central nervous system, causing confusion, poor coordination, and disturbed sleep patterns. While we could provide treatment for African sleeping sickness, there were no antiretroviral drugs available in South Sudan to suppress HIV. It felt completely hopeless not to have anything to offer.

This desperation was matched by a landscape in which there were no roads, no sanitation, and very little infrastructure, leaving the people at constant threat of disease. Even today, the life expectancy in Sudan is only 50. My work there not only made me appreciate what I have, particularly my education, but it also ingrained in me that I need to share my gifts with others, particularly those living with HIV.

For nine years now I have dedicated my life to fighting HIV/AIDS. It is like being on the front lines of war. While it does not kill with bullets or bombs, shrapnel or soldiers, HIV/AIDS is no less of an emergency. Where I live and work, AIDS is a crisis that claims thousands upon thousands of mothers, husbands, daughters, and brothers every year, without remorse or compromise.

Two million people lost their lives in 2007 because of AIDS, and millions more followed in 2008. Thirty-three million more are living with HIV. This is an epidemic that has spread like wildfire. In 1990, there were approximately eight million people with HIV/AIDS, roughly a quarter of what it is today. Sub-Saharan Africa houses two-thirds of the world's HIV-positive. In 2007, 1.6 million of the 2 million AIDS deaths were in sub-Saharan Africa.

In 2002, I left South Sudan for my home in Kenya to start an HIV/AIDS program with the IMC in Nairobi's Kibera slum. With more than one million people, Kibera is Africa's largest slum and has an HIV prevalence rate that is staggeringly higher than that of the rest of Nairobi. At that time, there were no antiretroviral drugs available in Kenya, so many of the people I provided services for were very sick, bedridden, their bodies depleted from the virus.

While I could not cure their HIV, I could still provide basic medical care for some of their ailments or take them to the hospital if they needed more advanced care. I spent each day visiting patients in their homes, making sure that they were as comfortable as I could make them.

Their physical pain was matched, if not exceeded, by emotional anguish. The presence of HIV/AIDS in the household created a myriad of emotional issues. Most were consumed with thoughts of the future, what their children and spouses would do after they died.

I knew from my experience that most of my patients just wanted someone to listen to them. Even if I could not give them anything else, I could make my patients feel valued and respected after feeling ostracized for having HIV. All it took was a simple conversation with someone who cared to help them overcome their hopelessness and find some salvation within themselves.

I became engulfed in so much heartbreak that I found it hard to separate my work from my personal life. Many of my patients started to call me at home wanting to talk. I had created a space where they could share their feelings and what they were going through, but many started to become overly dependent on me. I began to feel drained, exhausted, and emotionally stretched.

Drawing my boundaries was stressful, but I had to restore my personal health so that I could be fully engaged with those who relied on my support. I was taking care of about 300 HIV-positive patients who needed medical and emotional attention, and could no longer do it on my own, so I trained others in the community. This helped me find myself again in the midst of caring for others.

Later that year, we began another program in Kibera to prevent the transmission of HIV from mother to child. While the program was well received, we found that it was much easier to give women advice on breast-feeding than it was to actually get them to act upon it at home. This is mostly because of the dangerous stigma that exists around HIV/AIDS, as many women never tell their husbands that they are HIV-positive for fear of being abandoned.

In Africa, when a woman discloses that she has HIV, her husband usually leaves her, often for another woman. HIV-positive women are typically blamed for infecting their husbands or children, leaving them without family or even a way to support themselves. This stigma makes it incredibly difficult for a woman to tell her partner that she is HIV-positive. As a result, men often insist on having more children, creating a great risk for the virus to be passed on to the baby.

To overcome this stigma, we began educating the community about HIV and what it means for a woman who is pregnant. While it was not easy, our intervention had a 93 percent success rate, meaning only 7 percent of the women we worked with transferred HIV on to their babies.

We also created support groups where HIV-positive women could come together and find encouragement in one another. In my work, I have found that being a woman in Kibera is hard enough. For those with HIV, life is even harder, as they often do not have anyone to take care of them. These women need somewhere they can find relationships that do not vanish because they have HIV. That is what I try to provide for the HIV-positive women of Kibera, someone they can come back to time and time again when they need someone to acknowledge them, to remind them that they deserve to be listened to.

The fight against AIDS is far from over, but I found that one of the biggest weapons against this disease is women's empowerment. Whether or not they want to use a condom, have sex, or have a child, these are all choices that women cannot make for themselves. Their husbands and those around them make life choices for women. When a woman cannot decide what is best for her, she cannot protect herself from HIV or come forward to tell her partner that she is positive.

I hope to someday create a foundation where women can come to learn skills that will enable them to support themselves, with or without a husband or relative. If a woman is able to support herself, she can make healthy decisions and be the leader of her own life. I believe that if we can make more women empowered, we have won a critical battle in the war against AIDS.

This is something that I hope to instill in my daughter, Joy, now 15 years old. I sometimes take her with me to Kibera so she can volunteer. I am a single mother and support Joy and her 7-year-old brother, Dan, on my own. The two of them go to school in Nairobi. Martha is still an important part of my life. We often meet for coffee and share the latest updates on our lives.

I am now so attached to Kibera that if I have not been there for a week, I feel as though something is missing. My work in Kibera continues to be challenging, but it has also been deeply satisfying. This comes from feeling you have touched someone's life every day, that you have encouraged someone who has been discouraged, rejected, and discarded not for something they have done, but because they have HIV. I feel that just by listening I have given many a renewed reason to live.

Today, I no longer think about my scars or feel self-conscious about my appearance. I have been healed through helping others, caring not about my own scars, but about erasing the scars of others.

Preview

Caring Beyond Borders: Nurses' Stories about Working Abroad

~

Nancy Leigh Harless, ARNP

Coming in April 2010

Waterlife

~

John B. Fiddler, RN, ANP

EASTERN CHAD, JULY 2007: I find myself standing in a sandy clearing on the edge of what looks like a lake. The water is diluted chocolate milk. Across the water on the far bank, I see women and children wading and washing clothes. Behind them a gentle slope leads up to a village of traditional grass huts and the white tarpaulins of refugee shelters. Our land cruisers have just emerged from a grove of palm trees, and two rafts of empty oil drums lashed together are anchored to the bank and sit waiting. Above, birds with curved beaks circle and call. Our two cars are parked, spattered with drying mud, the engines clicking as they cool down after the journey. We can drive no further. This *wadi* is impassable and will be from now until November; we are all just glad to have made it this far. The waters are rising fast and we have to make the crossing without delay. Our destination: Kerfi, a bustling market town 45 kilometers south of Goz Beida, the regional capital of the Ouaddai province which forms part of the border with Sudan.

Watching us is a crowd of boys and some men. The boys seem to be smaller than their American counterparts for their ages, which I guess to be from 6 to 13 years old. Most regard us with some curiosity but generally appear unimpressed by our arrival. They are thin but strong and healthy looking. Their skin is patterned with dust or slick from the water. Some are chewing on the kernels of a coconutlike fruit from the palm trees that when split open reveals a bright orange pulp. This splash of color in a semi-desert landscape makes for an unforgettable first impression. Momentarily for me, the year 2007 ceases to exist, the ancient African past and the present become one.

It is hot here. So for six months of the year the waters become a cooling playground for these children. The water serves also as laundry, toilet, and garbage disposal and is often the only water available to drink. It is also home and breeding ground for some of the most insidious illnesses we will encounter, including the great killer, malaria. Our arrival noted, the kids resume playing and swimming. As we set off on the slow-moving rafts for the far shore, the boys dive-bomb us from the trees, laughing and screaming as they attempt to wet us. Today they are invincible.

Chad is my second assignment with Doctors Without Borders. I worked in Burundi for ten months in 2005, and there were no *wadis* there. Up to this point, I have only read about these riverbeds and hollows that are easily crossed on foot in the dry season, then turn to impassable milky torrents during the rainy season. Now I am going to spend most of the next six months surrounded on all sides by them.

Around Kerfi the local population converges on the town every Wednesday for a sprawling market that serves as a center of commerce and community. On market day, visitors will also take the opportunity to seek medical care. The village has a well-constructed, but barren, clinic manned by four government staff. They are minimally trained as health aides. There are no doctors. My role here then is multifold. I am tasked to supervise the facility and assist the government staff with training and teaching.

Our team also brings essential medications and will establish a pharmacy program. I will run a nutrition program and coordinate primary healthcare needs for a diverse population, including an influx of internally displaced persons (IDPs) forced from their homes close to the border with Sudan. These IDPs are the victims of new and old tribal conflict and ongoing war and are the main reason we have decided to establish a presence here.

In the rainy season, sickness here increases, mortality increases, and anyone seriously ill is effectively trapped. I look at the village looming closer and ask myself "what on earth am I doing here?" I am thousands of miles from New York City and my 21st century Critical Care Unit with high-tech modern equipment and fully stocked shelves. I'm used to having experts and laboratories just a call away. Will I be able to provide high quality care here with the limited resources? Will I be able to use my assessment skills as a new nurse practitioner? How will I be able to diagnose exotic diseases that I have only seen in books? I realize the answers will surely find me. I won't be going anywhere for a while.

There is no situation quite as overwhelming for a medical caregiver as encountering your first crowd of waiting patients in an African clinic. The majority are women and children, almost always accompanied by a chorus of babies crying. These are the most vulnerable and are also the first ones to sicken. I am nervous beginning my first triage rounds, walking through the assembled patients seeking those particularly ill who need to be seen first. Any child or adult with a fever (a cardinal sign of malaria) is automatically chosen and tested with a paracheck. This finger-prick test is rapid, and specific for malaria. If positive this is immediately an indication for treatment.

In every new field assignment, I learn to negotiate situations so that the sickest patient is cared for first. I soon learn that in Kerfi, a sick baby or mother is not necessarily a priority. Triage does not quite apply as I understand it. One soon realizes that the local tribal chieftain or the local military commander (and there are many of each) may take priority. Men also expect to be seen immediately and are uncomfortable waiting with females. We have to find a way to satisfy this population or no one will come to the clinic. We settle on the idea of making two separate waiting areas, one for women and children, the other for men. We triage women and children first, and then sit with the men and consult with them. We alternate between each group. This seems to work!

One particular tribal leader, swathed in a turban and dark glasses, walks into the clinic, pulls up his robe, turns his ample buttock towards me, and motions for an injection even though we have not even diagnosed an illness. Apparently, he had received an injection some time before and liked the result. I learn that many in the community see injections as an efficacious, almost magical treatment. They do not think tablets or oral medications really work. I realize that I am being taught unexpected lessons. To try and address the misinformation and rumors, I must organize community outreach and education. I learn too that some patients who receive prescribed medicine take all the tablets at once. Perhaps they think it will work better? After my initial surprise that they are still standing ("you took all 20 of the pills I gave you at the same time?"), I plan to do teaching at the pharmacy to help ensure better understanding and compliance.

Apart from women, crying babies, and pushy chieftains, there is another population that presents at the clinic that intrigues me: the same age children I see swimming at the banks of the *wadi*. They are mostly young boys, but a handful of girls. They wait hesitantly and shy, eyes held to the ground. Through an interpreter, I learn they have nonspecific symptoms, such as abdominal pain or nausea. My colleague who is familiar with schistosomiasis, a waterborne infection endemic among children in this part of Africa, teaches me the critical diagnostic question to ask these patients: what is the color of their urine? Almost always uncomfortably, they reply "pink." We have our diagnosis. Another lesson learned. The parasite that infects the children is contracted from the water while swimming, it eventually anchors in the bladder and produces a hematuria—blood in the urine. This disease can progress and can lead to serious chronic illness as the children grow up. If they grow up.

I grow sensitive to these patients. As a result, our team develops yet another simple parallel triage system. We put aside the children until there is a group of six or more. Then we take them together to be weighed and registered. The children stand in a line, traipse into our pharmacy room where they each take a one-time dose of Praziquantal medicine, and trot off into the distance. Most surely to swim and play in the microbe-laden water again.

These children quickly learn my name. As I walk the path back to our base at day's end, now no longer shy, they shout out "Jon, Jon, Jon!" to grab my attention. In the clinic, the colorful, chaotic crowds of mothers and babies demand most of your attention. The older children are already considered the survivors; they have made it past the vulnerable times and have hopefully developed a protective immunity to some diseases. You tend to regard them as invulnerable, as perhaps they do themselves.

One day at the clinic, I get a call to one of the consultation rooms to see a sick child. He is about ten years old. He is lying on a crude bed frame close to the ground. Beside the bed, his mother is on her knees holding his hand, mute with worry. The boy is breathing erratically, moaning, unresponsive and drooling, his eyes rolled back in his head. We are pretty sure he has cerebral malaria, a nurse pricks his finger to test—already we are putting in an IV. I demand a quick history of his illness: "Has he been sick long?" The translator tells me he had been playing and swimming the day before. We attempt to inject some dextrose to correct hypoglycemia (low blood sugar) and even as we try to save him, I know it is too late. Pink foam starts pouring from his mouth. It looks like someone has shaken a bottle of cherry soda inside of him. It's the ominous sign of pulmonary edema. Increased pressure in the blood vessels of his lungs has forced fluid into the air sacs, preventing them from absorbing oxygen. One of the nurses cautions me not to tell the mother her son will die—as is my nursing instinct—"this is not done here." So I stand there and watch him dying, as his mother sits beside him distraught. I have never felt so helpless. Time stands still in this moment as an African future is slowly extinguished.

That night, other members of our team and I go to bed extra-early before the mosquitoes begin their hungry dance at dusk. I wrap myself in my mosquito net and close my eyes. The bright color images of turbans, smiles, grimaces, and lives reel past. In America I have often heard it said that it is not natural for parents to outlive their children; it is not natural for parents to bury their own child. I write in my diary, "What do they know? It happens here all the time."

Four hundred and ninety seven days later in New York City, the images of the hundreds of patients we served daily still dance brightly in my mind. I save the most tender feelings for those boys and girls—full of laughter—swimming in the waters of the *wadis*, then shyly presenting for treatment at the clinic. The survivors. The invincibles. I wonder what the future holds for them? I wonder how they are now and has anything changed? Then I realize—I have to go back. I still hear them calling my name. They have more to teach me.

A Danish Nurse in China

~

Jytte Holst Bowers

"THE AMERICAN CONSULATE is looking for a nurse. Why don't you go for it?"

My friend Frances took my arm as we walked across the campus of Zhongshan University in Canton as she asked this question.

"Oh, no, dear friend. I've finished with that career long ago."

"Well, I just thought it a good idea. Think it over, won't you?"

I pondered for a couple of days, talked it over with Jim, my husband who had brought me to Zhongshan University where he and Frances taught English, and where I, together with other spouses, tried the almost impossible task of learning Chinese. At least in the job at the consulate I would be able to speak English, but I wouldn't remember much from my education as a registered nurse in Denmark over 30 years ago. Yes, I had had some retraining in the United States and worked as a nurse at the college where my husband taught, as well as in nursing homes in Michigan, Colorado, and South Dakota, but a nurse for the U.S. Consulate? That was somewhat doubtful.

A couple of days later, I hurried through the campus to catch a ferry across the Pearl River to a street in the inner city which was only a few blocks from the consulate in the Dong Fang Hotel. I wasn't the only person on that early morning ferry.

It was early April 1989. A dozen students also walked up the gangplank. They wore white headbands covered with Chinese characters and were searching their pockets for change. Their leader said something to the woman who collected the fares. She shook her head firmly.

"What is this all about?" I turned to a student in the hope that he could speak English.

"Well," he said, "we don't have money. We also pay for lunch. In Beijing busses let protestors go for free. All students free go to Tiananmen for democracy. Today we also go on march to show friends we care."

"I see," I said, "I'll take care of your fares." I gave the woman the few coins needed. When we reached the other side of the river, they joined the thousands of young people preparing their peaceful march toward freedom. I walked among the masses of Chinese on the street and reached the consulate just in time for my interview.

My first day at work was not a good beginning. The consulate had invited the doctor, an overseas Chinese woman, who was supposed to be my backup, and me to a banquet to celebrate our new association.

"Where is Dr. Ye?" I asked anxiously, sitting at a beautiful lunch table where nothing was missing but the doctor.

"You haven't heard? She is on her way back to America. She has a blood clot in her leg, and they thought it best she be transferred back to the states."

"Oh!" was all I could say as I dropped a delicious Chinese tidbit into my lap. So there I was, all alone, with no one to guide me.

"But you can always call the American doctor at the embassy in Beijing if you have any questions," he said.

No doubt the doctor was a very capable man, but did the consulate not know how inadequately the Chinese communication system worked in the Year of Our Lord 1989?

Nevertheless, I set up my office and prepared myself for my first patients. The nurse from the embassy in Beijing came visiting, and I received a welcome telegram from the ambassador. I was assured by everyone I would be fine. No one in the whole world can be more confident than Americans.

"Don't worry," the nurse from Beijing said, "just have your book on nursing procedures standing on a shelf in the bathroom. If you are in doubt, excuse yourself and go to the toilet, research the problem, and find the answer." Then we went to the market to find a teapot so I could brew myself a cup of tea, like the British nurse at the consulate in Hong Kong, which was close to Canton, but not yet a part of the mainland. Over tea all the world's problems would be solved.

The employees of the consulate were almost all young people who enjoyed a TGIF (Thank God It's Friday) at the end of the week. Their illnesses were of small concern: colds, headaches, diarrhea—much like those of the college students I had nursed ten years earlier. But after the visit of Surgeon General Dr. C. Everett Koop, the consulate had been anxious to find a hospital sterile enough to meet his demands—in case of an emergency. That was almost impossible to find in China only ten years after the end of the Cultural Revolution. Yet, when you visited the wards reserved for party members or foreigners, you might be impressed by how spotless they appeared to be. The nurses' uniforms were so white and starched they looked like crinoline. But the nurses did not realize that after a needle was inserted intravenously, it had to be taped down securely, among other things. As for the hospitals devoted to ordinary Chinese, they were simply filthy.

The emergency came on June fourth. At 2:00 A.M. I was called to the phone in the lobby. *Dear God, let it not be the American Consulate telling me the consul has had a heart attack*, I whispered to myself as I left our tiny two-room apartment at Zhongshan University.

It wasn't. It was my husband Jim's mother screaming into the phone all the way from Connecticut. "You have to come home, I am telling you. You have to come home. They are burning them. The busses are burning. The people are burning. You have to come home!"

The students who had gathered at Tiananmen Square for the last months had been attacked by the Chinese army. Some of those students were from our university and had traveled to Beijing to show their solidarity with their fellow students. My husband had gathered his graduate students in our apartment when he taught them a course in American literature. One of them had been the leader of the nightly marches out of the front gate of our university and into the city to join the young people from the other colleges in the city. We would never forget the day that young man quoted, quietly, but with determination, "Give me liberty or give me death."

Jim and I, indeed all Americans, including the women and children of the consulate, were ordered to leave China within 48 hours. My two months' work for the American Consulate came to a quick end. I folded my white jacket and went in to my boss.

"Good-bye and thank you," I said as I shook his hand.

"Yes, but you will be coming back when all this has blown over, won't you?" he asked.

"I doubt it. This has been too much for my husband and me, but thank you once again."

In 2005 we returned to China to teach for one semester. I assisted Jim by helping small groups of students to practice their spoken English.

"Why did you leave China when you seemed to have liked it so much?" they asked.

"We left because of Tiananmen," I answered.

Their faces were blank. Later I learned from Jim's Chinese colleague that the Chinese government had rewritten history: the massacre on Tiananmen Square never occurred. No one is allowed to speak about it. The younger generation knows nothing about the students who sacrificed their lives to the Goddess of Liberty. But on this 20th anniversary, we are lighting a candle on the evening of June fourth and placing it in our window in their memory, for we have the freedom to express the sorrow we have felt over and over again—to act on behalf of our Chinese friends who do not have that freedom.

In the Doghouse

~

Fiona MacLeod, BSN

In JULY OF 2008, looking for a bit of adventure, culture, and travel, I left my comfortable research job in Vancouver, British Columbia, and set off to the Middle East. I had accepted a one-year contract working on a ward at a large research hospital in Saudi Arabia. Little did I know at that time, that these 12 months were to be the most significant learning experience of my entire life to date, culturally, professionally, and personally.

One of the most significant things I have learned is just how powerful language can be. Making the effort to acquire and use even a limited vocabulary of the local language can create bonds and help to seal off deeply running cultural fissures.

Often, my narrow berth of the Arabic language limits me to using words that I know aren't exactly right in a particular context, however in most situations, the point usually gets across and my faltering attempts are generally met with encouragement and endearment. My efforts also provide much needed comedic relief for both the patient and myself within the sober hospital environment.

Every day, I am adding to the list of words that I keep in my pocket, and every night, I try to practice each one and commit it to memory. I am proud to say that I can now ask any Arabic-speaking patient if they have moved their bowels today, yesterday, or the day before yesterday, whether they have had any diarrhea, whether or not they are constipated, and if they would like any medication to assist in whatever dysfunctional bowel pattern they may be experiencing. Unfortunately, this wealth of knowledge does not transfer well to communication with the general public, such as at shopping malls or with cab drivers, etc.

I should also make clear that, at the beginning, while I could get a basic point across, I generally spoke either in very short sentences with devastatingly poor grammar or in single words punctuated with animated gesticulations to get my point across. The latter method was not always well received before I learned all my bowel-related Arabic.

My first language blunder happened in the first week on my new ward. First, a bit of background: though the holy Qu'ran emphasizes kindness to all animals, dogs are considered "dirty" in Islam. Muslims do not keep dogs as pets in Saudi, and generally the only place one can see a dog is a fleeting glimpse of a wild *saluki* in the desert. Touching a dog voids *wudu*, the ritualistic washing of one's self with water prior to each of the five daily *salas* (prayers).

One of my first proud new words was *gelb* which means "heart." The "G" sound in Arabic is quite soft, and can almost be mistaken for a "K." On one particular day, I was happily doing my morning assessments in my patients' rooms. When it came time to use my newly acquired vocabulary, I would lift my eyebrows, point at his/her chest and say *kelb*? as in "can I listen to your heart?" By the third patient, I could not shake the feeling that I was getting a little bit of hostility, although I told myself that it was a cultural thing that I was no doubt misinterpreting.

It wasn't until later on that day, when I was practicing my Arabic with one of my Lebanese coworkers, that I realized my embarrassing blunder. Apparently, I had been pronouncing my "G" sound *too* softly, and it was coming out as a fairly audible "K." While *gelb* means "heart", unfortunately *kelb* means "dog." In case there was any doubt as to whom I was referring when I uttered the insult, I must remind you that I pointed at my patients' chests while saying it. As an aside, I also found out later that single-finger pointing at someone in any capacity in the Muslim culture is also insulting. Oh dear—strike two.

My Arabic has come a long way since this first incident, though not without additional and equally amusing blunders. Though I am proud to say that I have developed a fairly good "working knowledge" of the language, I am also aware that in certain situations, it is not appropriate to have any ambiguity around what is being said. In some instances, the necessary explanation or command of the language goes far beyond what I am capable of.

A very important lesson I have learned is that sometimes, just staying completely silent while doing your job quickly and expertly speaks louder and more articulately than the most intelligent and thought-provoking exchange in *any* language. In keeping with this, I would also like to share a more recent experience with language.

One of my patients was scheduled for a bone marrow biopsy. If you have ever experienced either receiving, observing, or assisting with a bone marrow biopsy, you know well that "barbaric" is a gross understatement in describing the procedure. The patient lies in a semi-prone position while the doctor drives a needle, roughly the width of a chopstick and the length of your hand, from wrist to tip of your baby finger, through layers of dermis and muscle, and into the bony pelvis. The intention is to collect a corkscrew-like sample of bone marrow to analyze for blood cancer.

I say "intention" because often, it takes more than one trip of boring the needle through the fleshy tunnel and retracting it to check if the sample attempt was successful. This procedure is done under local anesthetic and a needle as long as your middle finger filled with xylocaine is driven into the flesh and alternately eased forward and backwards to ensure that an adequately wide area has been numbed. The patient gets some premedications for pain and for anxiety, but I liken this to offering someone a Tylenol and a lavender oil neck massage before a bilateral leg amputation.

This particular patient had a history of chronic pain and depression, and was particularly anxious and teary prior to and during the procedure. I pulled up a chair beside her bed and held both her hands, as I spoke in my best soothing voice and tried desperately to pass on strength and will to the distraught woman. The woman cried out in pain and clamped my hands in a diaphoretic vice-grip as the needle drove into the back of her pelvis.

The doctor who was performing the procedure is an incredibly intelligent man, meticulously conscious of minute details "behind the scenes." Unfortunately, however, his bedside manner would no doubt cause Florence Nightingale to have a serious nervous meltdown. He is not a native Arabic speaker but seemed to truly believe that knowing how to say "Is there pain here; you are not feeling pain; and what is the problem?" in Arabic was an acceptable range of vernacular to competently perform this procedure.

As these questions were delivered in his signature manner with a harsh, accusatory "Huh?" after every question, I felt my jaw clench tighter and tighter as the patient's cries grew louder. My "Western-style" temper erupted violently over the edges of the gender-repressed container I had packed it into, for the time being, in order to assimilate into my new culture.

His third, "There is not pain; what is the problem? Huh?" was cut short by my urgent, even statement, that surprised even me as it quietly but forcefully escaped my lips.

"With all due respect, doctor, I think the crying and the yelling is fairly indicative of the pain, and the problem is that she has an eight-inch needle the size of a pencil stuck into her pelvis. Can we just get this over with as quickly as possible, please?"

The room was suddenly silent except for the whimpered Qu'ran verses escaping the pursed lips of the young woman. You could cut the tension with surgery shears. I calmly and firmly met the Doctor's patronizing stare, despite the creeping fingers of crimson that slowly made their way up my neck and pricked my ears.

Just when I was certain that the doctor was going to stalk out of the room leaving the biopsy needle protruding out of the patient's pelvis like a Saudi oil rig, he broke the gaze, muttering something about protocol. The remainder of the procedure was slightly tense, but thankfully quick, quiet, and relatively uneventful.

Experiences like this one taught me that gaining a handle on the local language is essential, but it is not enough. It is just as important—even a professional responsibility—to know our limitations, use sound judgment, and be honest about the range of our abilities, both to ourselves and with others.

Acknowledgments

"Fronting up to a Civil Emergency," by Julie Vickery, is reprinted with the kind permission of the journal *Kai Tiaki: Nursing in New Zealand*, October 2004.

Reader's Guide

1. As a depth psychologist, Mark Montijo in "Hunting the Lion That Swallowed You," believes that if we discern meaning from traumatic events, we may be able to contextualize it within our lives in a way that makes sense and creates a new and stronger order. Do you think this possible? How can we do this in order to achieve lasting and positive life changes?

2. Have you ever been faced with making a decision that could have a positive impact on someone else's life but could put you in mortal danger, as LeAnn Thieman describes in "How Did I Get Myself into This?" How did you respond?

3. In "Sleepless in the Sahara," one can almost see the resettlement camp, feel the wind, taste the grit, and experience the author's frustration when the water trucks don't arrive. Many tales from disaster health-care workers speak to the need for the survivors to tell their story. Discuss the importance of the disaster workers themselves telling their story and having it heard as a form of self-care.

4. In "Fronting Up to a Civil Emergency," Julie Vickery speaks of her role as the emergency team leader. What do you see as her greatest strengths during the Manawatu floods? Similarly, in his story of flooding in a major medical center, Chad Ware manages his hospital's Emergency Department's complete evacuation plan and implementation. Does your workplace have a disaster plan? What is your role in case of disaster?

5. In times of disaster, many are joined in a united effort to overcome adversity and bring back a sense of normality to their country and fellow man. Describe some of the events that demonstrate pride and self-sacrifice in the stories you've read.

6. In "Bent but Not Broken," the author finds that in the midst of the rubble of Hurricane Katrina, she is surrounded by positive, upbeat people. From an elderly coworker nun to a Southern gentleman who serves coffee on china he scrounged from the debris, she is touched by their optimism and sense of hope. Discuss what you think allows people to feel hopeful in the wake of destruction and loss.

7. Christine Tebaldi speaks of learning the skill of "compassionate presence" in the essay "The Day My World Started Turning Faster." What does this mean? Have you had the opportunity to experience compassionate

presence with a patient, client, friend, or family member? If comfortable, please share your story.

8. In "There Is a Way from Heart to Heart," Dr. Goodman mentions that the Afghans' "physical ailments were paired with psychosocial pain." Discuss this concept and the importance of providing holistic care—treating the whole person rather than simply the symptoms.

9. In "Tsunami!" Marko Cunningham reports that he worked in the disaster recovery for several weeks without a break. Speak to the need to balance self-care with the push to get the job done during a disaster. Can these same concepts apply to any job?

10. Have you ever found yourself in an emergency situation where you were forced to adapt, like Ronda M. Faciane in "Go with the Flow, Adapt to the Changes"? How did you manage?

11. In "Angels on the Battlefield," medical supplies are running dangerously low and soldiers are being wounded every day and require surgery. The head nurse asks two corpsmen to risk their lives to obtain needed medications and supplies for the wounded soldiers. Discuss this ethical quandary. Does the end justify the means in time of war or other disasters?

12. In "The Day of the Great Wave," Perry Prince uses a
     tube of sunscreen as a ritual "talking stick" to encour-
     age each member of the group to have his story heard.
     What is the value in this? What are other rituals that
     help us deal with grief and loss?

13. Discuss the Chinese people's openness to the Trauma
     Resiliency Model (TRM), presented in "Trauma,
     Healing, and Serendipity in the Sichuan Province,
     China." Compare and contrast this model to a more
     traditional model of psychotherapy. Do you think
     that a culture of Eastern medicine would be more,
     or less, open to this model than a culture of Western
     medicine? Defend your response.

14. Grace Muthumbi in "Beauty and Grace" and Mark
     Montijo in "Hunting the Lion That Swallowed You"
     write about the physical and emotional demands that
     service to others in emergency situations entails. How
     do these demands affect your spirit and body? What
     can be done to protect yourself spiritually and physi-
     cally to prevent burnout so that you can still be of
     service to others?

About the Editors

NANCY LEIGH HARLESS is a woman's healthcare nurse practitioner who worked with the International Medical Corps in the post–Balkan War recovery effort. She is also an award-winning poet and writer. Her poems and stories have appeared in many anthologies, including *Lyrical Iowa*, *Traveler's Tales*, *Cup of Comfort*, *The Healing Project*, *Chicken Soup for the Soul*, and Kaplan's own *Nurses' Voices*, as well as in many professional and literary journals. She is the author of *Womankind: Connection & Wisdom Around the World*, a collection of short stories based on her international nursing experiences and travels.

Now retired, Nancy lives in Iowa with her husband, Norm, but travels often—usually off the well-paved road.

KERRY-ANN MORRIS lives in St. Andrew, Jamaica, and is employed as the information officer at the Office of Disaster Preparedness and Emergency Management (ODPEM). In that capacity, she is responsible for satisfying the disaster information needs of the Jamaican public through the development and implementation of public education and public relations programs in keeping with the mandate and functions of the organization. During periods of emergencies, Kerry-Ann serves as the media liaison arm between the ODPEM's National Emergency Operations Center in Kingston and the national and international media.

Kerry-Ann is the author of *Living Well with Endometriosis: What Your Doctor Doesn't Tell You...That You Need to Know.*

About the Contributors

SCHARMAINE LAWSON-BAKER would probably plead guilty to having a missionary zeal for her clients. She is the CEO of Advanced Clinical Consultants, a network of home-visiting healthcare providers. A native of New Orleans, her path to a home healthcare NP practice started while she was pursuing her degree at Tennessee State University, where she joined humanitarian mission trips to the Dominican Republic and Puerto Rico. She has recently started a nonprofit agency, Geriatric Initiatives, and just finished her Doctor of Nursing Practice degree from Chatham University in Pittsburgh, Pa. in August of 2008.

RENEE BERKE is a registered nurse who studied with Planned Parenthood at The New Jersey College of Medicine and Dentistry in Newark, and practiced in Boston as an ob-gyn nurse practitioner. She presently lives in Cape Cod and has written for *The Barnstable Patriot*, *The Cape Cod Times*, *Advance for Nurses*, and other nursing periodicals. In 1999 she volunteered as a national disaster nurse with the American Red Cross.

SANDRA (SAM) BRADLEY has spent 30 years as a para-medic, field supervisor, educator, and writer. She is a self-proclaimed "disaster junkie" and has been the train-ing officer for the federal Disaster Medical Assistance Team, CA-6, for about 10 years. She has published arti-cles in EMS magazines, written for textbook publishers, and participated in several disaster exercises in Ukraine. When she isn't training new EMTs or firefighters, she's working on the next "Great American Novel."

MARKO CUNNINGHAM is a New Zealander working in Thailand for a Thai NGO for nine years now. Marko works mostly as an EMT, but he also takes care of the dead, teaches volunteers, and helps distribute relief sup-plies all over Thailand. During the Tsunami of 2004, Marko helped take care of 2,500 bodies at Bang Muang Temple in Southern Thailand. A book on his life called *Sleeping with the Dead* will be published this year (*www.bkkfreeambulance.com*).

RONDA M. FACIANE was born and raised in New Orleans, LA. She graduated from LSU School of Nursing with an associate's degree in 1991 and her bach-elor's degree in 2000. She is the mother of two children, Alexis and Marc. Ms. Faciane is currently employed by the Overton Brooks VA Medical Center in Shreveport, LA. She resides in Greenwood, LA, with her husband Eddie and son Marc.

LINDA GARRETT has a BSN from the University of Delaware. She has been the school nurse at Laurel Springs School since 1999 and has worked as a staff nurse on the inpatient Child/Adolescent Psychiatric Unit at Kennedy Hospital since 1993. She was certified as a psychiatric/mental health nurse in 1996 and has been a Red Cross volunteer since 2001. She is married and lives in southern New Jersey.

DR. JEFFREY C. GOODMAN, a retired family practice physician from Kauai, has served as a spokesperson and volunteer field physician for International Medical Corps (IMC) since 1987. He has been with IMC on ten different missions, many of them emergency response, in eight different countries, including Pakistan, Afghanistan, Sudan, Iraq, Liberia, Indonesia, Lebanon, and Kenya.

DIONETTA M. HUDZINSKI has over 40 years' nursing experience in a variety of healthcare settings including ten years as clinical instructor at Washington State University, and over ten years as a clinical nurse consultant for pain and palliative care. Dionetta volunteers for a chronic pain support group and is a member of the Clown Ambassadors of Yakima, WA. She learned her clown skills from a Shriner clown and hospice patient after bringing his pain under control.

RHONA KNOX PRESCOTT recently retired to Skaneateles, New York. She finished nursing school in Flushing, New York, and was commissioned in the U.S. Army in the Nurse Corps. She served for approximately seven years, one of those in Vietnam during the Tet offensives of 1967 and 1968. After the war, Rhona completed a master's degree in clinical social work at the University of Houston and eventually became a trauma counselor/therapist for war veterans. She writes for publications now, and some of her work has been adapted for stage. Busy as a mom and grandma, life is good. Volunteer work keeps her grounded and happily occupied.

ELAINE MILLER-KARAS is the codirector and cofounder of the Trauma Resource Institute. She lectures internationally about integrative healing approaches for treating trauma and has cocreated the Trauma Resiliency Model (TRM). She has worked in Thailand, California, New Orleans, Baton Rouge, and Africa. She co-coordinates the Chinese Earthquake Relief Project, which is cosponsored by the World Health Organization in China, training Chinese doctors, nurses, counselors, and teachers in TRM. She is also working with survivors of the May 12th earthquake.

MARK A. MONTIJO grew up on a horse ranch in Southern California. Now living at the base of Mount Diablo in Northern California with his wife and three daughters, Mark divides his time between working as a healthcare ombudsman/mediator for a large HMO and teaching as an adjunct faculty member at Pacifica Graduate Institute in Carpinteria, CA. In his spare time, Mark enjoys reading, writing, and mountain biking with his family.

GRACE MUTHUMBI has served as a health worker and HIV/AIDS activist with International Medical Corps (IMC) for nine years. She first worked with IMC in South Sudan, where she was involved in a Center for Disease Control and Prevention study on the co-infection of African sleeping sickness and HIV. A native of Kenya, she later returned with IMC to lead a new HIV/AIDS program in Nairobi's Kibera slum, where she still works today.

PERRY PRINCE has worked in disaster mental health since 1997, serving with the American Red Cross to assist in 17 disasters, including 9/11, Katrina, and typhoons in U.S. territories in the Western Pacific. He has also worked on international assignments with other NGOs: in Sri Lanka, following the tsunami that is the subject of this story, with Sri Lankan refugees in India, and most recently, in Uganda, where he did an extensive psychosocial assessment of Congolese refugees.

RICK RHODES retired from the Army National Guard in 2007, after 16 years of active duty service in the United States Army and 4 years with the Florida Army National Guard, and was deployed in Operations Desert Storm and Iraqi Freedom. He worked as a terrorism planner for the Florida Division of Emergency Management and was assigned to the state's Emergency Response Team-A. As regional emergency response advisor for the Florida Department of Health, he responded to several natural disasters, including Hurricanes Charlie, Frances, Jeanne, Ivan, Katrina, Rita, and Wilma in 2004 and 2005. Currently, he holds a position with the Department of Veterans Affairs as an area emergency manager.

ROBERT B. ROBESON flew 987 combat medical evacuation missions in South Vietnam. He had seven helicopters shot up by enemy fire and was twice shot down in one year. He was commander and operations officer during his tour with the 236th Medical Detachment (Helicopter Ambulance) in Da Nang. He is a writer who has been published more than 700 times in over 250 international, national, and regional publications, which include *Reader's Digest*, *Official Karate*, *Vietnam Combat*, *Sepia*, *Executive Female*, *Frontier Airline Magazine*, and *Newsday*, among others. He has garnered a readership of millions in 130 countries. He's also a member of the National Writers Association and the Military Writers Society of America. Robeson retired from the U.S. Army as a lieutenant colonel, after 27½ years of military service on three continents.

LOUISE M. ROBINSON earned her RN degree at the age of 45, then joined the Peace Corps and was sent to Guatemala, where she single-handedly enriched the lives of an entire country. Certified as an International Red Cross volunteer nurse, she was sent to Kuwait to assist at a refugee camp. Louise continues to do volunteer work while working as a registered nurse in Colorado. Raising her grandchildren has been only one of her many adventures.

SALLY ROY-BOYNTON received her MSN from the University of Dubuque and her doctorate in business administration (DBA) from California Coast University. She is a certified nursing executive and a clinical specialist in adult psychiatric nursing. Ms. Roy-Boynton is Director of Psychiatric Services at Mercy Medical Center, Dubuque, IA. She does volunteer work as a disaster mental health counselor for the American Red Cross and is active in the community, where she serves on several agency boards.

CHRISTINE TEBALDI is a psychiatric mental health nurse practitioner with a specialty in Emergency Services and Disaster Mental Health. She completed her nursing education and began her career at the University of Rochester. Currently, she holds a clinical and administrative position at McLean Hospital. She has held several leadership roles with the American Psychiatric Nurses

Association. Ms. Tebaldi is an active member of the American Red Cross, as well as a disaster mental health instructor.

LEANN THIEMAN is a nurse, author, and member of the Speaker Hall of Fame. Believing we all have individual "war zones," her keynotes and seminars motivate health-care givers to balance their lives, live their priorities, and make a difference in the world. She has been featured in *Newsweek*, PAX-TV, FOX-TV, NPR, and PBS. She is coauthor of ten Chicken Soup for the Soul books, including *Chicken Soup for the Nurse's Soul* and *Chicken Soup for the Caregiver's Soul*.

JULIE VICKERY lives in Palmerston, North New Zealand, and is the charge nurse of the MidCentral Health District Nursing Service. This service provides intermediary care, linking primary and secondary services. This service is free of charge to all patients. Julie's passion for nursing involves achieving the best possible care for patients on their journeys through primary and secondary services, through excellent coordination and communication. Julie is married and has three adult children.

CHAD WARE has been involved with emergency management and disaster preparedness since 2001. He is a member of Iowa's Federal Disaster Medical Assistance Team, IA-1. He has responded to Hurricanes Katrina, Rita, and Ike, and he participated in the Health and Human Services response to New Orleans. Chad's most recent disaster experience occurred at home with the Iowa Floods. Chad assisted in coordinating the successful evacuation of 183 patients when the floodwaters reached the front doors of Mercy Medical Center in Cedar Rapids. Chad has worked as an emergency department nurse and currently holds the position of emergency management coordinator at Mercy Medical Center, Cedar Rapids, Iowa.